Biostatistics With 'R': A Guide for Medical Doctors

Marco Moscarelli

Biostatistics With 'R': A Guide for Medical Doctors

Springer

Marco Moscarelli
Department of Cardiovascular Sciences
GVM Care & Research, Maria Eleonora Hospital
Palermo, Italy

ISBN 978-3-031-33072-8 ISBN 978-3-031-33073-5 (eBook)
https://doi.org/10.1007/978-3-031-33073-5

This Springer imprint is published by the registered company Springer Nature Switzerland AG
The registered company address is: Gewerbestrasse 11, 6330 Cham, Switzerland

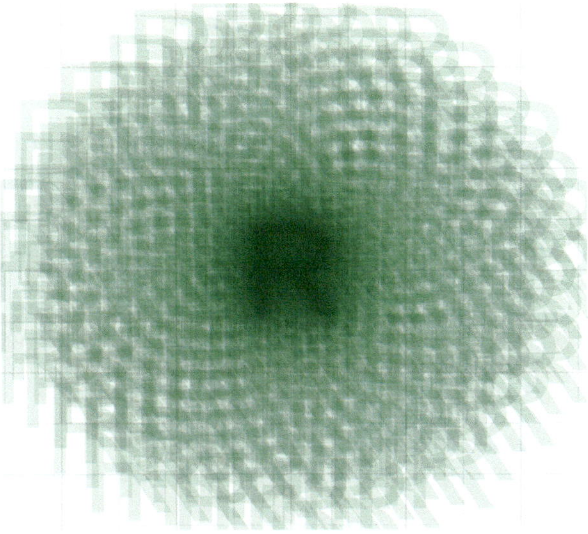

Foreword

It is indeed my pleasure and privilege to write the Foreword for the textbook entitled: *Biostatistics with "R"- a Guide for Medical Doctors*. I had the privilege to work closely with Dr Moscarelli in several diverse research projects where he made significant contributions to the development and understanding of biostatistical concepts.

This book contains all the essentials of biostatistical principles, methods, handling of variables and health statistics that constitute an essential foundation for everyone interested in these subjects.

I am pleased to recommend this book for every medical and health professional and for all those who are interested in establishing practical biostatistical skills.

The vision of this book is to provide pillars for both biostatistics and coding with "R". R is an exciting statistical package that offers all standard and many advanced methods of data analysis. In addition, general methods such as linear and logistic regression have extensive capabilities for the analysis of survival data, longitudinal data, and complex survey data. For all estimation problems, inferences can be made based on more robust calculating capabilities of statistical uncertainty measures which are significantly enhanced by a team of excellent statisticians and developers of R commands. R is extremely powerful, is easy to use through its intuitive command syntax. All research community finds R a rewarding environment for manipulating data, carrying out statistical analyses, and producing publication quality graphics.

This book is the starting point for professionals who want to acquire advanced knowledge in statistical methodology. The topics are broad, but it is important to explore them. All are crucial biostatistics components, which anyone wanting to write and/or truly understand any scientific literature. Also, such topics will help the reader to sharpen his/her scientific mind and better formulate research questions. A clear, original research question is the foundation of a solid scientific paper which also needs to be assessed as better as possible with the appropriate methodology.

Cardiovascular Sciences and Cardiac Surgery
Imperial College London,
London, UK

Thanos Athanasiou

Preface

The strange image on the cover page represents the two-dimensional fractal nature of the "romanesco" broccoli in a very simplified way.

This vegetable is the most intriguing paradigm of fractal geometry. The broccoli is the result of layers of spirals, each layer arranged intentionally at a "golden angle". The science that studies how plants arrange their leaves is called "phyllotaxis".

Plants grow in a structured and non-chaotic way, mainly in order to maximise their exposure for photosynthesis while reducing stress. The golden angle is defined by the formula $\pi(3 - \sqrt{5})$, and this number is inspired by the golden ratio, one of the most famous numbers in the history of mathematics. The image on the cover page and others which appear at the beginning of each chapter were generated using "R".

It would be interesting to understand how such fractal patterns can be observed in humans. Nevertheless, this book is about biostatistics, so let's not diverge from that.

This book *Biostatistics with "R": A Guide for Medical Doctors* is structured as a scientific journey of sorts. All statistical explanations and examples in this book are based on a fictitious, yet potentially true, dataset named `MMstat`. It contains data from fictitious groups of patients who undergo cardiac surgery. One of the groups has administered a "high broccoli dietary regimen" sometime before surgery. The other control group is not. We are interested in understanding whether the group administered the broccoli, with its anti-inflammatory properties, might experience improved post-operative outcomes after surgery. The dataset contains figures from the pre-operative period ("*baseline patients' characteristics*"), the operation ("*operative details*") and early and post-operative outcomes ("*follow-up*").

In this book, analysing the example dataset `MMstat` provides the ability to discuss the basic principles of biostatistics with the aid of "R".

"R" is not just a software for statistics, but an environment capable of generating images like the one on the cover page of this book. Explaining biostatistics requires images and graphics since visualising data "brings data to life".

"R" is one of the most powerful environments for data visualisation. By the end of this book, you should be able to scrutinise any dataset, describe a population, perform hypothesis testing, and analyse results.

Why is this relevant for medical doctors? In practice, we are not able to understand any scientific papers or discuss them critically, if we do not have a solid biostatistical foundation. How does one define a p-value? What does odds ratio mean? What is the difference between odds and probability? Or between linear and logistic regression? What is a "goodness of fit" of a regression model? As doctors, we are surrounded by graphics, survival curves, forest plots, and many other data visualisation tools. This book aims to teach you, not only how to interpret such data visualisation tools, but also how to construct them, with the help of "R".

Palermo, Italy Marco Moscarelli

Contents

Chapter 1
Introduction

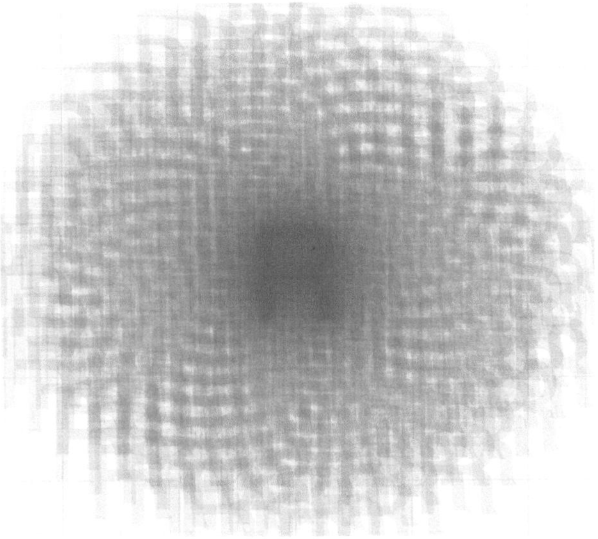

1.1 Introduction

There is only one way to learn “R”, download “R” (and “R-studio”, which makes life simpler) and start typing. Simply type anything and you will learn by doing. Well, probably you will need a helping hand, but the message is that you need to practice using “R”, a lot!

M. Moscarelli, *Biostatistics With ‘R’: A Guide for Medical Doctors*,
https://doi.org/10.1007/978-3-031-33073-5_1

There are, in fact, many ways to learn biostatistics. One of them is by using "R". You may think "R" is complicated, since you must learn not only statistics but also coding to use it (for "R" to function, it requires a language based on codes). But learning the code and using "R" will help you immensely in understanding and presenting biostatistical information.

This book is about using "R" and biostatistics to analyse scientific data and is tailored for whoever works in the medical field. Learning the fundamentals of statistics, and also how to code with "R", will make you a better scientist and perhaps a better doctor.

Nevertheless, both "R" and biostatistics are in all respects more complicated than the topics covered in this book. The vision with this book is to provide pillars for both biostatistics and coding with "R". You may be stimulated to acquire more advanced knowledge further down the track, but this is the starting point.

This book covers many concepts of biostatistics, with some emphasis on visual data representation. It has a practical component, and it comes with a dataset called "`MMstat`" which is downloaded from "GitHub", a repository website. More explicit instructions of how to download the dataset are set out in Chap. 2. The example dataset is fictitious but contains potentially realistic information (including baseline patients' characteristics, operative details and post-operative outcomes) of patients who undergo cardiovascular surgery.

1.2 What Is the Dataset About?

When I was studying in London for my post-graduate degree, a colleague was conducting a study for his PhD. The study was to investigate the influence (if any) of broccoli extract given orally to patients before surgery and the inflammatory response in the post-operative period. While the outcome of the study is unknown to me, the idea intrigues me.

Alongside this book, the fictitious dataset `MMstat` was created solely to provide an example for the purpose of this book. The fictitious dataset simulates data about two groups. The first control group consume a liberal diet pre-surgery. The second group carry out a high broccoli dietary regimen pre-surgery. The "MM" from `MMstat` represents the initials of my first name and surname.

Throughout this book, any coding and all variables from the dataset included in "R", along with functions and objects created in "R", will appear in the following format:

```
> MMstat<- 'this is my dataset'
```

Data was fictitiously created in excel and saved in .csv (comma separated value) format. The example dataset can be downloaded from GitHub:

https://github.com/mmlondon77/Biobook.git.

The dataset MMstat contains all relevant data including the baseline patients' characteristics, operative details and post-operative outcomes.

This book will step by step outline the statistical analysis required to answer a research question. In the case of the example dataset: does including the high broccoli dietary regimen pre-surgery improve post-operative outcomes?

By scrutinising the dataset, the baseline patients' characteristics and subgroup differences are investigated, graphics are created and a statistical hypothesis is formulated. Finally, the research question is examined and answered.

1.3 What You Will Learn

The figure below represents the work/study flow of this book (Fig. 1.1):

In particular you will learn:

i. How to download and install "R" and R-studio
ii. How to perform the basic, yet relevant coding required to use it
iii. How to import a dataset and start data exploration with some more advanced R-coding
iv. About subsetting with "R" as well as advanced data subsetting
v. About ggplot2 (the grammar of graphics), an additional R-package
vi. How to check for normality before further analysis as well as more R-coding, subsetting and data visualisation for both numerical and categorical variables
vii. About central tendency as well as the mean, median, mode and measure of spread (variance and standard deviation) of a dataset
viii. About correlation and more on data visualisation and subsetting for correlation
ix. About hypothesis testing and how to create tables for a research paper
x. About regression, linear regression, logistic regression as well as a small amount of non-linear regression
xi. About survival analysis and Cox regression
xii. How to control for confounders and the basics of propensity score matching

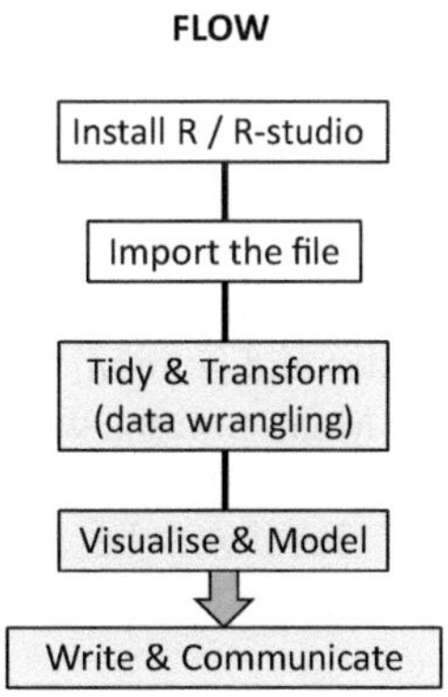

Fig. 1.1 Work/study flow of this book

The topics are broad, but it is important to explore them all. All are crucial biostatistics components, which anyone wanting to properly write and/or truly understand any scientific paper needs to master. Also, such topics will help you to sharpen your scientific mind and better formulate research questions. A clear, original research question is the foundation of a solid scientific paper.

If you are new to statistics, and especially to “R”, it is strongly suggested that you read all chapters of this book in the order set-out.

1.4 Why This Book?

Because it is written by a medical academic doctor (myself) to another medical doctor (yourself). We know our limitations but also our ambitions.

Importantly, by reading this book you *will neither* become a statistician *nor* a data scientist. For more comprehensive biostatistics, you should consult a trained biostatistician. However, by mastering the content of this book, it will become easier for you to interact with any biostatistician or data scientist, because you will learn to “speak the same language”.

Knowledge is communicated in a practical way throughout this entire book, by analysing the dataset `MMstat` as if it is a real patient scenario.

At the end of the journey, you will better be able to produce a full statistical analysis, with tables and plots, ready to start assembling a scientific paper. You will master data wrangling and manipulation, data normality checking, hypothesis testing, regression and survival analysis. In order to minimise the confounders, you will understand how to perform propensity score matching.

The process requires a lot of willpower and effort from you. But at the end of the day, it will be rewarding and you will stand out from the crowd.

1.5 How This Book Works

Because the book is designed to work alongside the dataset `MMstat`, every chapter comes with associated “scripts” that can be downloaded along with the .csv format of the `MMstat` dataset.

These can also all be downloaded at GitHub:

https://github.com/mmlondon77/Biobook.git

By downloading the dataset and launching the scripts, you can reproduce the codes and generally all the graphics and figures provided in this book.

Many notions will be repeated at different levels and in different chapters. This is done purposefully to make it easier for you to digest all concepts.

There will be a little algebra, but any essential formulas are provided and discussed.

1.6 What Is "R" (and R-Studio)?

I won't spend much time describing what "R" is and why "R" stands out above other software. Few words are needed!

"R" is a programming language and free software (or better: "environment") developed by Ross Ihaka and Robert Gentleman in 1993. "R" is open source and cross-platform compatible (it can be installed on Windows, MAC and Linux). "R" provides a variety of statistical techniques and graphical capabilities. Importantly: "R" has countless extensions (named R-packages), for a range of applications.

This book will enable you to construct your knowledge on "R" step by step and layer by layer. Some concepts will be hard to understand at first glance, especially some of the R-coding or advanced plotting with the grammar of graphic R-package. Hence, some topics, along with their relevant coding, will be given at different levels and will be repeated with many examples throughout the book. In fact, "R" can be used at different levels with different potential.

To set a foundation, provided below are two different sets of original figures (Figs. 1.2 and 1.3) produced with two different systems of graphics.

The first picture (Fig. 1.2) was obtained using the "basic graphic" function in base-R. It is a simple four-panel figure that requires a very long and demanding code. Every single detail in the figure had to be entered with line code and took a long time to build. The research was published by my group in the European Journal of Cardio-Thoracic Surgery (Moscarelli M, et al. Remote ischaemic preconditioning in isolated aortic valve and coronary artery bypass surgery: a randomised trial. Eur J Cardiothorac Surg. 2019 May 1;55(5):905–912) where data was analysed (troponin and cardiac metabolites) from patients who had ischemic preconditioning before surgery.

Whereas the second picture (Fig. 1.3) was created using an R-package, specifically grammar of graphic (`ggplot2`). It refers to a more recent study published in EHJ-Quality of Care and Clinical Outcomes that meta-analysed several quality-of-life (QoL) domains after coronary bypass surgery at different time points (Creber RM, Dimagli A, Spadaccio C, Myers A, Moscarelli M et al. Effect of coronary artery bypass grafting on quality of life: a meta-analysis of randomized trials. Eur Heart J Qual Care Clin Outcomes. 2021 Oct 13:qcab075). On the left side the values are represented as "spaghetti plots", on the right side as "weighted box-plots".

This research is not discussed here, neither is the code which built Figs. 1.2 and 1.3. It is simply to demonstrate the huge graphical potential of "R" that spans from very basic graphics to complex and colourful images. I personally believe that Fig. 1.3 is more valid, yet it requires a shorter code. For example, note the differences between the boxplots in Figs. 1.2 and 1.3. The latter has "jittering", meaning it has a number of observations depicted in a single boxplot.

In a dedicated section of a chapter of this book, `ggplot2`, the package used to construct Fig. 1.3, is explained in more detail.

Important advice and things to note about "R":

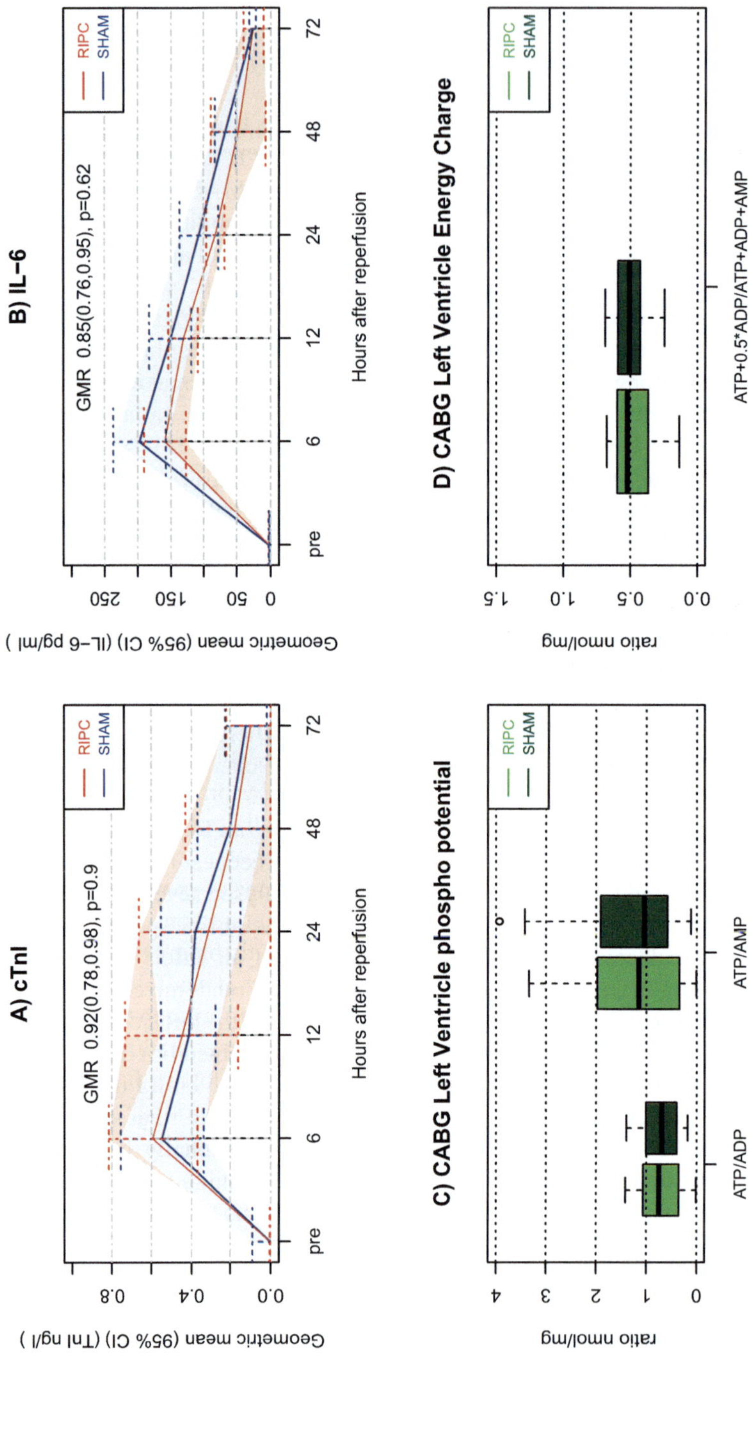

Fig. 1.2 Four-panel figure produced with "basic graphic" in "R"

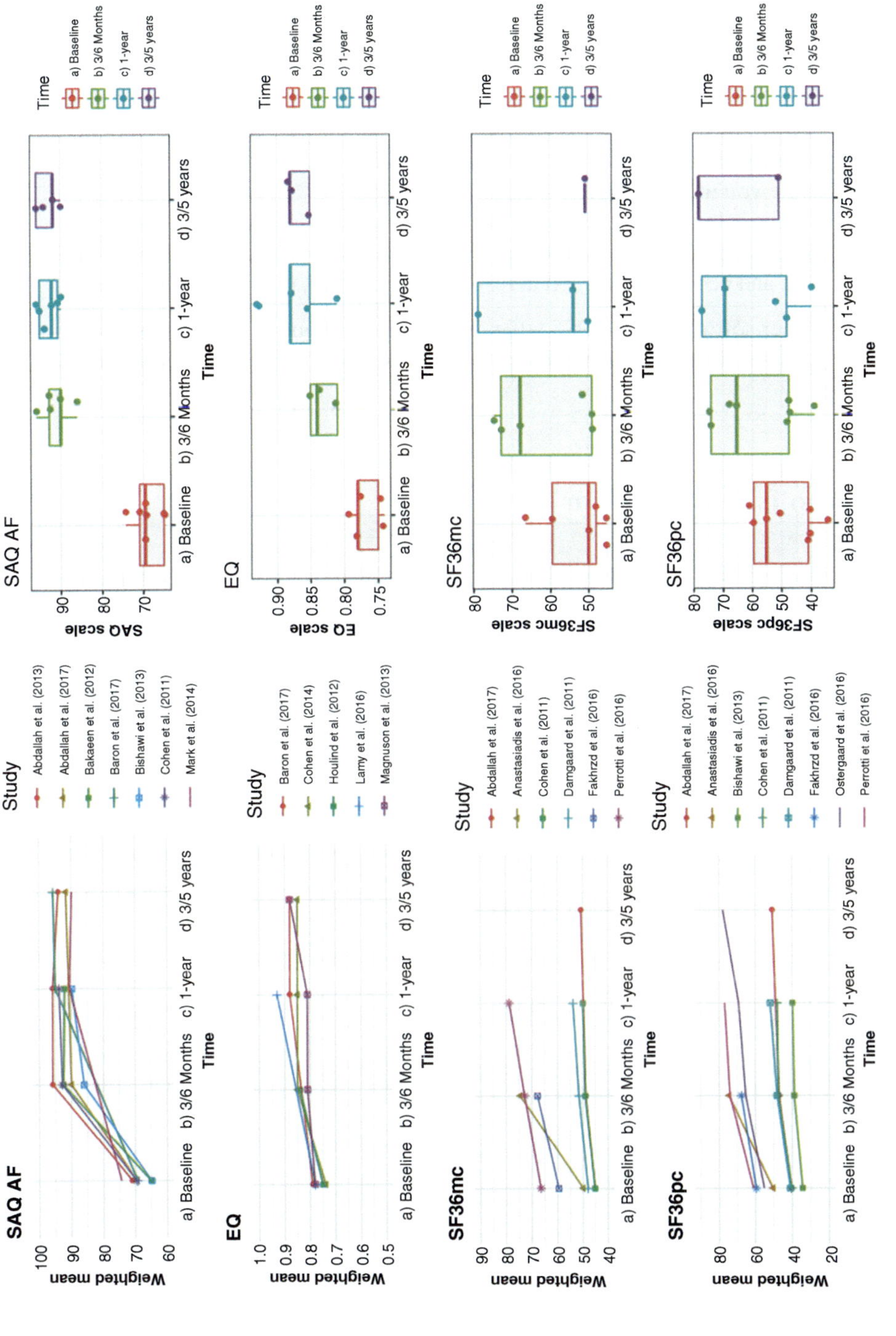

Fig. 1.3 Advanced plotting in "R" using the additional R-package ggplot2

1. To learn how to successfully manipulate and present biostatistical data using "R", you must be strongly motivated. You will encounter many obstacles, as per any complex learning.
2. "R" is very picky (and sometimes painful). Even a misplaced comma will corrupt a code. In fact, at the beginning, you will often end up with many wrong codes that result in error. "R" is specific! With practice you will get better, coding will be easier and it will become easier to detect and correct any errors you make while you are coding.
3. Perseverance is key; do not abandon "R". "R" is a booming language and worth the effort to learn it. If you want to perform solid statistics, create well-performing figures and become published in respectable journals, then "R" is the answer.

Unlike other software (e.g. SPSS), the analysis carried out in "R" is transparent and easy to share. In fact, it is based on code and scripts that can be passed on to other peers.

1.7 Who Is This Book For?

As suggested by its title, this book is mainly for medical doctors since the topic of interest is a medical concern and it talks about medical and surgical intervention.

If you already have a solid knowledge of statistics and R-coding, you may find this book too simple for you.

Nevertheless, anyone in the generic biomedical field, who wants to scratch the surface of biostatistics and R-coding, will indeed benefit from reading this book.

To reiterate, reading and practicing with examples in this book will *only* scratch the surface! Mastering proper R-coding requires extensive time and dedication.

"R" has a huge virtual Web-based community, eager to help. If you are stuck for any reason, any Web-based search engine will direct you to find answers to your questions.

Chapter 2
How "R" Works

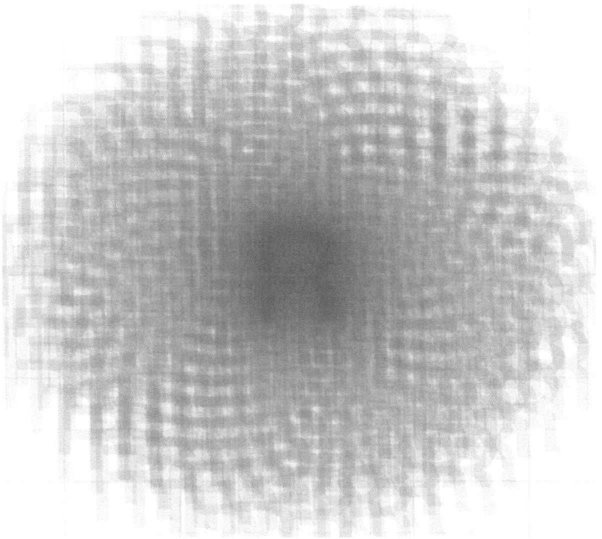

2.1 Downloading "R" and R-Studio

In order to start our scientific journey and perform our analysis, we need to install:

- "R" (base-R)
- R-studio

M. Moscarelli, *Biostatistics With 'R': A Guide for Medical Doctors*,
https://doi.org/10.1007/978-3-031-33073-5_2

Both are free.

You can download base-R at:

https://www.r-project.org

You can download R-studio at: https://www.rstudio.com/products/rstudio/download/#download

and follow the links.

Base-R is the basic software which contains the "R" programming language.

But why also R-studio? It is better to use R-studio because it is a more friendly interface in comparison to "R". However, to run R-studio, you must also have base-R ("R") installed on your computer. Using R-studio inside base-R is the recommended choice. In fact, all the coding and analysis presented in this book is done in R-studio.

2.2 What R-Studio Looks Like

When you open R-studio, it will look similar to below:

R-studio has a four-pane workspace. What I like to name each pane is set out below, alongside its corresponding letter from Fig. 2.1, together with a description of its function:

A = CODE EDITOR: allows you to create and open a file containing R-script. Basically, the R-script is where you can edit and store your work. You will soon download a script from GitHub to create your first plot.

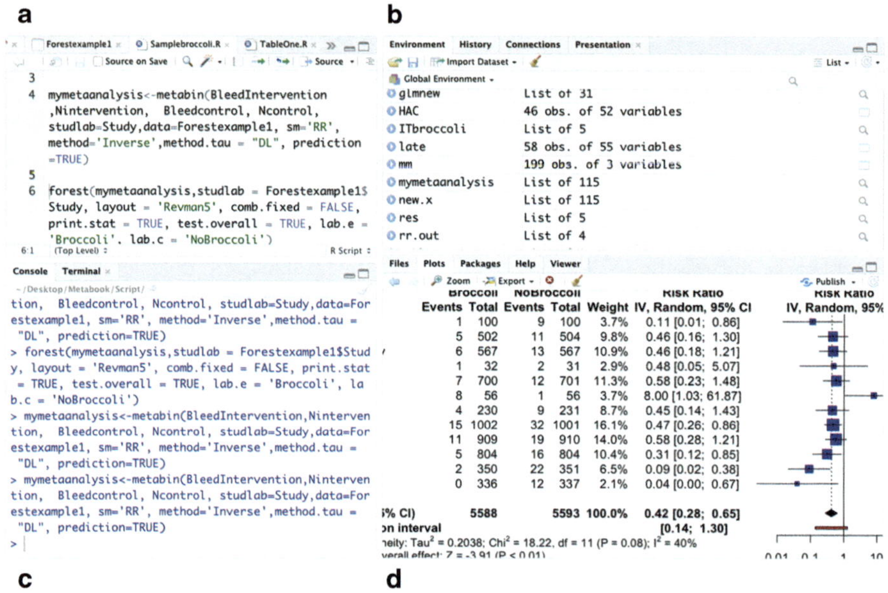

Fig. 2.1 How R-studio looks with the four-pane workspace

B = GLOBAL ENVIRONMENT also WORKSPACE and HISTORY: the environment tab shows the list of R-objects created during the R-session. The history tab shows the history of all objects created.

C = R-CONSOLE: where we can directly type and run our code, if preferred, rather than working within script.

D = PLOTS and FILES: under the packages tab is where you see which R-packages are installed (R-packages are a type of module or extension for doing certain things; this will become clearer when we work with different packages that allow us to perform specific analysis). The plots tab in this pane sets out all created plots. The help tab is also found in this pane.

2.3 Running Simple Codes in the "R"-Console

This section describes in very basic terms how "R" works, for any complete beginners to start immediately practising with the console.

To start, let's run an elementary code in the console as shown in Fig. 2.2:

```
> 1+1
[1] 2
```

> is the symbol for "prompt" which basically notifies the console to carry out whatever task follows the prompt symbol. Typing `1+1` in the console returned the sum of `2`.

Next, let's create an object as shown in Fig. 2.3:

```
> x<-1+1
```

Now, anytime we type `x` again into the console, it will return the sum of `1+1` equal to `2`.

The <- arrow is the "assignment statement" which assigns the elements which follow it. In this instance the assignment statement assigns `1+1` to the new object `x`. In this case the elements are numeric, but they can also be non-numeric. In this

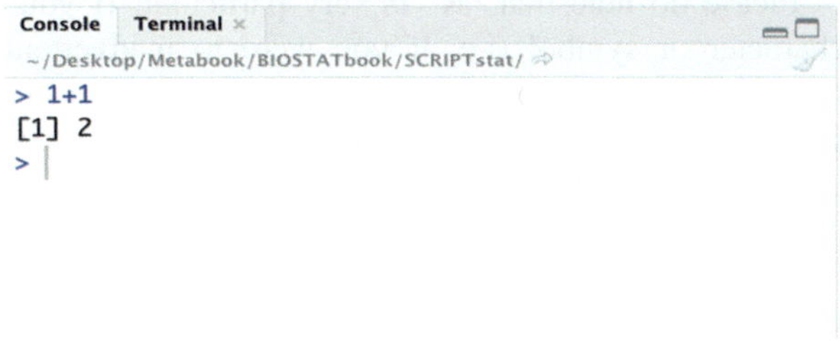

Fig. 2.2 Basic math in R

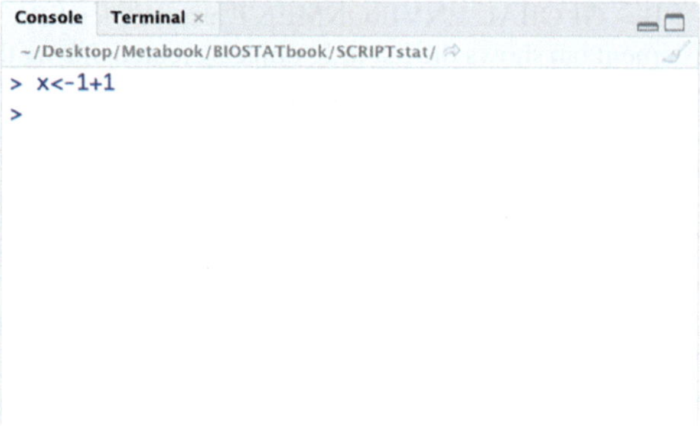

Fig. 2.3 Creating an object named "x"

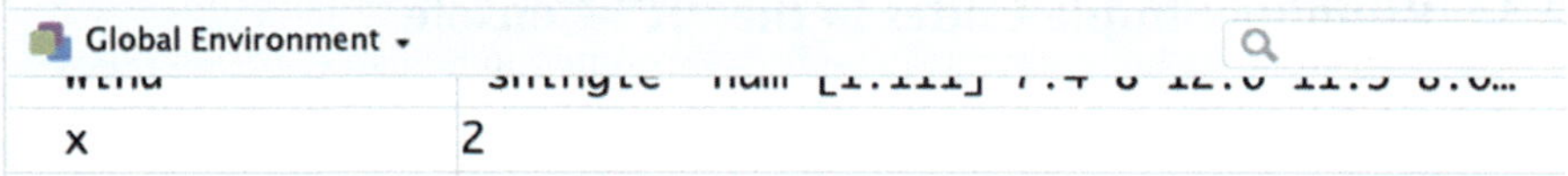

Fig. 2.4 The object "x" appears in the "Global Environment"

example, from now on (until the code may be modified with a new instruction), `x` will store the content `1+1`.

In the Global Environment (i.e. the top right pane of the four-pane workspace), the object will be created and stored as `x` (Fig. 2.4).

2.4 To Practice with a More Advanced Code

Let's assume that in my hypothetical surgical team, I have six fellows. I want to know the average height in cm of my surgical team. We collect the height of each team member and create an object that contains the heights of all six (the elements):

```
> height<-c(177, 167, 172, 174, 176, 178)
```

A new object is created, named `height`, and contains all six elements.

Note, the operator function `c( )` is also added to the code; this concatenates the elements (Fig. 2.5).

Please do note that "R" is very particular. If you forget or misplace a single character or symbol (i.e. if you were to inadvertently forget a comma in this example), it will return an error. Now, we have created the object `height` which contains the concatenated heights of all six colleagues, we can now go ahead and calculate the mean using the `mean( )` function:

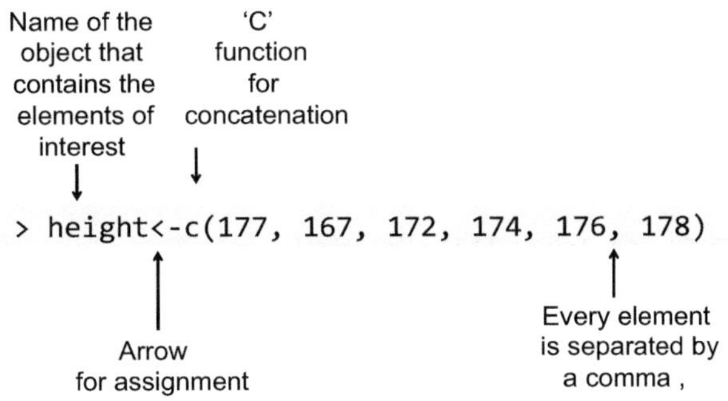

Fig. 2.5 Concatenated elements of the object "height"

```
> mean(height)
[1] 174
```

and "R" returns the sum of the six heights divided by six (174 cm).

We can now conclude that we have calculated 174 cm as the average height of my team. With these few lines we have already learnt how to create *objects* and use *functions*.

Everything in "R" is an object. We can refer to `height` also as an "atomic vector". Atomic vectors are simply vectors of data, in this example, the heights of my colleagues.

We can expand the atomic vector and assign names to it, as set out in the code below:

```
> names(height)<-c('Mark', 'Jessy', 'Frank', 'Robert', 'Andy',
'Maria')
> height
  Mark  Jessy  Frank Robert   Andy  Maria
   177    167    172    174    176    178
```

The function `names` includes the names within an object. Those are the fictitious names of my colleagues. How many elements does our vector contain? Let us expand our knowledge a little more about R-function and use the `length( )` function:

```
> length(height)
[1] 6
```

This function reveals our object `height` has six elements, being the heights of each of my six surgical peers. There are endless basic and advanced functions in "R" that simply cannot all be discovered here. But we will look at many of them in this book.

Notably at this stage, we have still not uploaded any dataset. So far we are simply creating objects in "R". Soon you will learn how to upload files and apply the same functions to the variables of a dataset.

2.5 Getting Help in "R"

There are two ways to find help for using "R". To provide an example, we reflect on the function `mean`:

```
> help(mean)
```

or

```
>?mean
```

When typing one of the two above commands into the console, the following information relating to the function `mean` will appear (Fig. 2.6) under the help tab in the lower right pane of the four-pane workspace (defined earlier as the PLOTS and FILES pane and labelled D in Fig. 2.1):

Another avenue, as specified in the introduction, is the solid Web-based community of "R". You can search the Web for any questions you have using any online search engine, and it will return the answer you are looking for.

mean {base} R Documentation

Arithmetic Mean

Description

Generic function for the (trimmed) arithmetic mean.

Usage

```
mean(x, ...)

## Default S3 method:
mean(x, trim = 0, na.rm = FALSE, ...)
```

Arguments

`x`	An R object. Currently there are methods for numeric/logical vectors and date, date-time and time interval objects. Complex vectors are allowed for `trim = 0`, only.
`trim`	the fraction (0 to 0.5) of observations to be trimmed from each end of `x` before the mean is computed. Values of trim outside that range are taken as the nearest endpoint.
`na.rm`	a logical value indicating whether `NA` values should be stripped before the computation proceeds.
`...`	further arguments passed to or from other methods.

Fig. 2.6 Finding help in "R"

2.6 The Hash Symbol

The hash symbol # is widely used in "R" for adding comments amongst code. Anything written within the same line of code after the symbol # is disregarded by "R".

```
> # after the symbol # R ignores what you write so you use # for
making comments and annotation
> #mean(height) # it does not return any action since after the
symbol # R ignores the function mean
```

This is very useful when we have a long script and code and we need to make annotations to help us remember and understand what the scripts are about. For example,

```
> names(height)<-c('Mark', 'Jessy', 'Frank', 'Robert', 'Andy',
'Maria') #Those are the names of my colleagues (this function is
especially helpful when the person entering the data is not the
only person viewing, using or analysing the data)
```

Notably, the text after # does not affect the capability of "R" to interpret the code. "R" simply ignores it. The code above is short, but when you have multiple lines, you need comments to better navigate and keep track of what level you are at.

2.7 The Problem of Missing Data

Missing data is very common in a dataset. Any missing data will appear as `NA` (not available). Missing data might heavily affect statistics. Some values might be missing on purpose, others by chance. Sometimes we may need to manually input missing variables, but that is beyond the scope of this book.

As a very simple example, let's assume that we do not have the value of the height of one of my colleagues as below:

```
> height<-c(177, NA, 172, 174, 176, 178)
```

The height of the second person is missing. When we try to calculate the `mean`:

```
> mean(height)
[1] NA
```

"R" does not know how to deal with missing values, which is why it returns `NA`.

To calculate the `mean,` we must tell "R" to remove or ignore the missing value as per the code below:

```
> mean(height, na.rm=TRUE)
[1] 175.4
```

The function `na.rm=TRUE` prompts "R" to ignore the `NA` amongst the values which is affecting the object height. This is most helpful when dealing with much larger datasets with missing values.

As you know, in medicine, it is common to handle such datasets with missing values.

2.8 Misspelling the Code

As outlined earlier, "R" is very exact. Every misplaced comma or misused capital letter will result in an error.

For example:

```
> Mean(height)
Error in Mean(height): could not find function "Mean"
```

this is because `Mean` is incorrect when entered with a capital M.

Another example of "R" being very particular is set out below:

```
> height<-c(177, NA, 172, 174 176, 178)
Error: unexpected '>' in ">"
```

The problem is highlighted in red. The comma which should naturally separate the two variables is missing, and "R" returns the code as an error. Again, when writing code with "R", one must be very precise, since even the slightest omission or error will affect results.

2.9 Setting the Working Directory

The working directory is the file path that indicates where all the files are saved in "R". It can be anywhere and can be modified according to your preference. I personally set my working directory, for the sake of simplicity, in a folder on my desktop. To know where the working directory is located, you may want to use the function `getwd( )`:

```
> getwd( )
[1] "/Users/marcomoscarelli/Desktop/Metabook/BIOSTATbook/SCRIPTstat"
```

This function returns the file path, and, as you can see, in this case it is in the folder `BIOSTATbook` on my desktop.

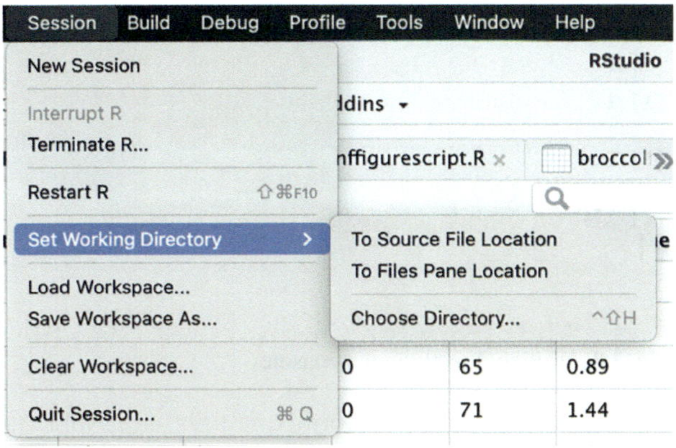

Fig. 2.7 Setting working directory

There are ways to change the working directory. The `setwd(dir=)` function can be used. But probably the easiest way is to use the menu as shown in Fig. 2.7:

2.10 Working with Scripts

What are scripts? Why are scripts so important in "R"?

There are two ways to write in "R". The first way is to write directly in the console. All the simple coding we've done so far was written directly in the console. This is specific for small and simple lines, like calculating the mean of a vector, or for simple algebraic operations like the one below (Fig. 2.8):

Writing directly in the console is great, but nothing will be saved. If we want to save our code, we must use a script. Scripts are also better when the code is long. In the case of an error, scripts help us to avoid starting all over again.

How to launch a script?

Figure 2.9 shows the quickest method:

A script is a series of codes, like the one shown in Fig. 2.10:

Note that in a script, unlike when writing directly in the console, you must tell "R" to run the code. There are a few ways to do that.

One of the easiest ways is to put the mouse cursor at the end of the code and click "run", as depicted in Fig. 2.11:

Alternatively, you can highlight the code you want to run first and then click run as shown in Fig. 2.12:

You may want to save a script (in .R format) in the working directory or wherever is more convenient for you.

You can store complex coding in a script that represents advanced statistics or plots. As outlined previously, you can share scripts with your peers. Once saved, you can email it, and when launched, it will open in the "R" environment.

Fig. 2.8 Writing directly in the console

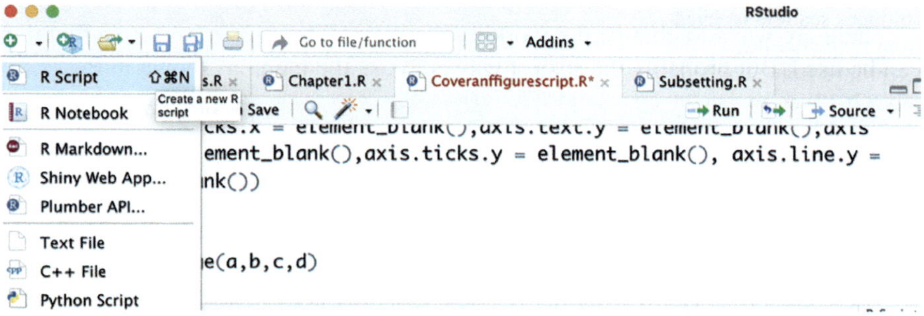

Fig. 2.9 Creating a script

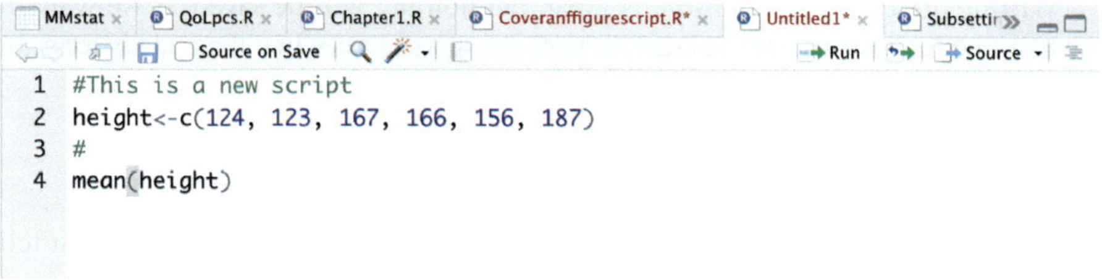

Fig. 2.10 Creating the script "height"

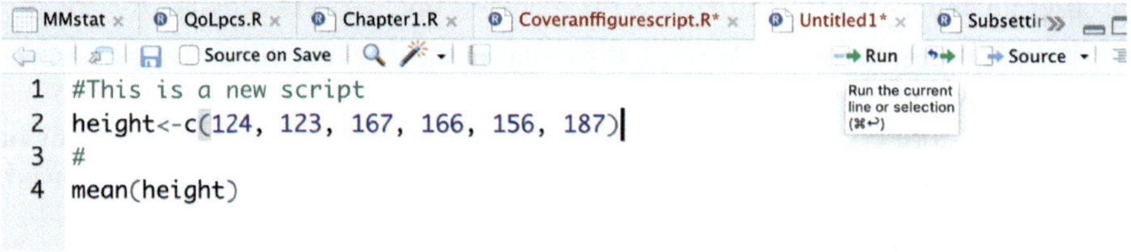

Fig. 2.11 Running the script with the cursor at the end of the line

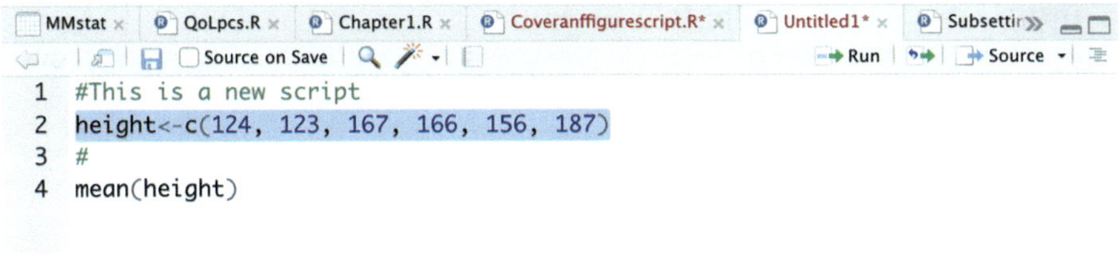

Fig. 2.12 Running the script with the code highlighted is another way

2.11 R-Packages

"R" comes with pre-installed base-R software. Base-R contains many functions that will be used on a daily basis (e.g. ones that we have already used in the paragraphs above, such as `mean( )` or `length( )`).

Base-R contains functions (the basic statistical functions) created by the original authors. But "R" is an open source, and many other authors have contributed with their own unique functions (creating R-packages).

A package is a bundle of data that includes functions/examples/help menus all included in an organised self-contained package.

In order to use a package, other than that already available in base-R, you have to *install* it. After installing it, you have to *load* it.

2.12 Installing R-Packages

To install a package (i.e. to download it) the `install.packages( )` function is used:

```
> install.packages('name of the package') # and we need to insert
between the brackets the package of interest that we would like
to install
```

By doing so we can download any R-package from the Comprehensive R Archive Network (CRAN). CRAN is the central repository for R-packages. Let's make an example. Let's assume that we want to download and install the package `corrplot`.

In the console, you should see the following message set out in Fig. 2.13:

The package `corrplot` is used later in the dedicated chapter about correlation.

Once installed, the package remains in the software memory, and you do not need to install it again. But after installation, you need to load it as shown in the following section.

```
> install.packages('corrplot')
Installing package into ‘/Users/marcomoscarelli/Library/R/4.0/library’
(as ‘lib’ is unspecified)

  There is a binary version available but the source
  version is later:
         binary source needs_compilation
corrplot   0.89   0.90             FALSE

installing the source package ‘corrplot’

trying URL 'https://cran.rstudio.com/src/contrib/corrplot_0.90.tar.gz'
Content type 'application/x-gzip' length 2820127 bytes (2.7 MB)
==================================================
```

Fig. 2.13 Installing a package with the “install.packages( )” function

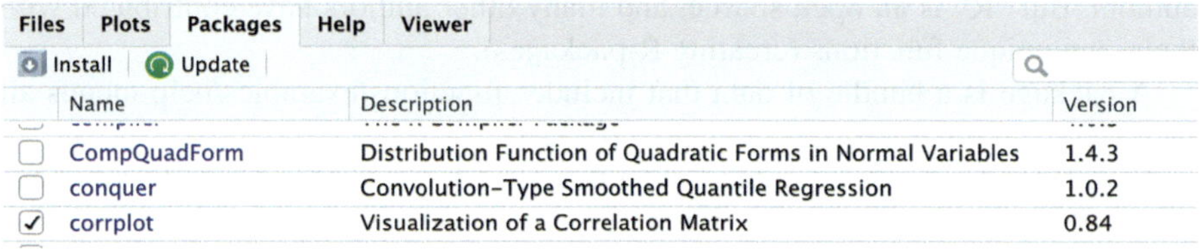

Fig. 2.14 Loading the library “corrplot”

2.13 Loading R-Packages

After installing, a package is almost ready to use. Next it must be loaded using the `library( )` function (Fig. 2.14):

```
> library('corrplot')
```

In the lower right panel of the four-pane workspace, you may double-check that the package is installed and loaded. When it is, you are now able to use all the functions of this package, which will be explored further in the dedicated chapter for correlation.

There is a potential shortcut, being the `package::function` function. Say we want to use a certain function from a package without loading it, we can use this function as a shortcut. For example, we would like to use the function `corrplot.mixed( )` from the package `corrplot` without loading the specific package; we must enter into the console:

```
> corrplot::corrplot.mixed()
```

Simply, we are prompting “R” to run the `corrplot.mixed( )` function only, from (`::`) the package `corrplot`.

This is a nice shortcut and can be used anytime. You simply need to type the package name along with the function required.

2.14 How Many R-Packages Do We Need?

There are endless packages in "R". You only need to install and load the packages relevant to your analysis.

We should be able to perform basic biostatistics with the pre-installed packages in base-R. Needless to say that all the packages are free. Further detail is provided later in the book outlining which packages are best used for specific types of analysis.

So far, you have been exposed to `corrplot` for correlation or `ggplot2` for data visualisation.

2.15 Conclusions

This chapter describes how to download "R", what "R" is, how it is composed and, most importantly, the vital basic "R" functions to start coding. It specifies that it is easier to use R-studio, since the interface is smoother and more intuitive.

Coding is immense and can take time to learn, especially for medical doctors, not primarily interested in data science. This chapter describes some very fundamental functions in "R" in the simplest possible way. Those are the foundation.

Later in the book, more advanced and somewhat complex functions will be demonstrated in more detail. It is made clear that "R" requires continuous learning.

Importantly, this chapter also describes the value of scripts, what R-packages are and how to install and load them. We will extensively make use of several R-packages throughout this book.

Further Readings

R Core Team. R: A language and environment for statistical computing [Internet]. Vienna, Austria; 2016. Available from: https://www.R-project.org/.

de Vries A, Meys J. R for dummies. Chichester: Wiley; 2012.

Wickham H, Grolemund G. R for data science: import, tidy, transform, visualize, and model data. 1st ed. O'Reilly Media; 2017.

Witten D, James G, Hastie T, Tibshirani R. An introduction to statistical learning: with applications in R. New York: Springer; 2013.

Chapter 3
Exploratory Data Analysis in "R"

3.1 Software and R-Package Required for This Chapter

If you haven't already, you need to download and install base-R and R-studio as set out in Chap. 2 under the heading "Downloading "R" and R-studio".

To carry out the exploratory analysis in this chapter, you will also need to download and install the R-package called tidyverse at the following link:

http://tidyverse.tidyverse.org

M. Moscarelli, *Biostatistics With 'R': A Guide for Medical Doctors*,
https://doi.org/10.1007/978-3-031-33073-5_3

3.2 Importing a Dataset into "R"

To download the supplementary dataset created as a practical example for use throughout this book, you need to find the file `MMstat.csv` at the following link:

https://github.com/mmlondon77/Biobook.git.

The necessary script for this chapter `Chapter 3.EDA.R` is also found at the link above.

When you download it, it is best stored in the working directory. As a reminder from Chap. 2, to locate or to change your working directory you may use the function `getwd( )`.

The following Fig. 3.1 shows how the file should look when you open it on the GitHub website:

As demonstrated in the following Fig. 3.2, to download the dataset, you should click on the green "code" button and from the drop-down menu click on "download ZIP":

Once you have downloaded the file `MMstat.csv`, I suggest you move it to your working directory.

Next, there are many ways to import the file `MMstat.csv` into "R". Probably the easiest one is the `read.csv( )` function in "R":

```
> MMstat<-read.csv(file='MMstat.csv', header = TRUE)
```

Importantly, `header = TRUE` is entered, which prompts "R" to read the first line as the headers of the columns. Remember from Chap. 2 that the file was originally saved in the format comma separated value (.csv). Remember also, as explained in Chap. 2, that if the file is not saved in the working directory, then you should specify in "R" the pathway to find the file.

Finally, we should visualise the dataset using the `View( )` function to start exploring the file:

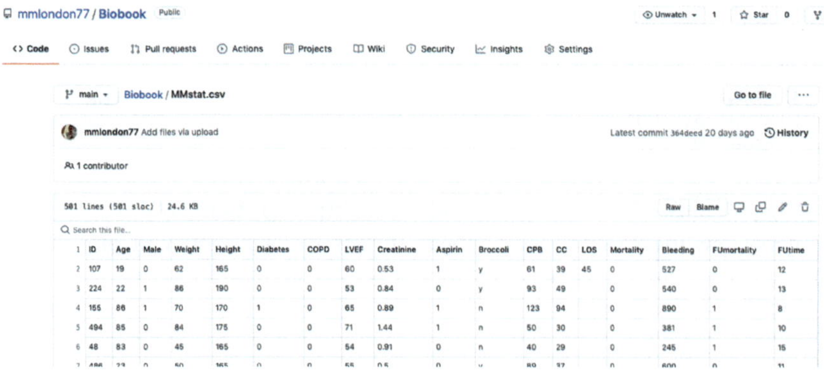

Fig. 3.1 A small screenshot taken from the GitHub website looking at the dataset MMstat

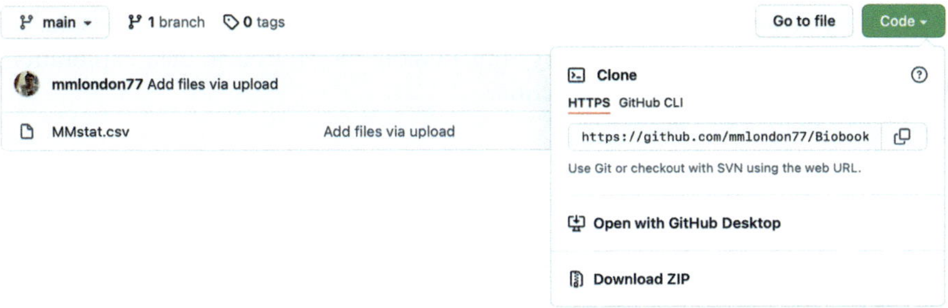

Fig. 3.2 Downloading the dataset MMstat.csv from GitHub

	ID	Age	Male	Weight	Height	Diabetes	COPD	LVEF	Creatinine	Aspirin	Broccoli	CPB	CC	LOS
1	107	19	0	62	165	0	0	60	0.53	1	y	61	39	45
2	224	22	1	86	190	0	0	53	0.84	0	y	93	49	NA
3	155	86	1	70	170	1	0	65	0.89	1	n	123	94	NA
4	494	85	0	84	175	0	0	71	1.44	1	n	50	30	NA
5	48	83	0	45	165	0	0	54	0.91	0	n	40	29	NA
6	486	23	0	50	165	0	0	55	0.50	0	y	89	37	NA
7	194	27	0	89	180	0	0	60	1.23	1	y	93	66	NA
8	140	83	1	70	163	0	0	51	0.81	0	n	50	20	5

Fig. 3.3 The dataset MMstat imported into "R"

```
> View(MMstat)# or view with lower case will do the same
```

You can see the result of this command in Fig. 3.3.

There are also other similar functions such as:

```
> read.table()
> read.csv2()
```

I reiterate from Chap. 2 that you can always ask for help with the `help( )` function (e.g., `help(read.csv)`).

3.3 Fundamental Function to Explore a Dataset

First things first. Once a dataset file is imported and you can see it in the top left pane of the four-pane workspace of "R", it is time to ask several questions. How many variables does it contain? What are they called? How many observations are there? How many rows and columns are there? Finally, what kind of variables does the dataset contain? In fact, you should also scrutinise the dataset for missing observations.

See an example from dataset `MMstat` below:

The figure above shows how the dataset `MMstat` will appear in the console.

There are many pivotal (and easy) functions in "R" for basic data exploration. We will start with the `dim( )` function:

```
> dim (MMstat)
[1] 500  18
```

"`dim`" stands for dimension, and it returns how many rows and columns a dataset has. As set out above, the example dataset has 500 rows and 18 columns.

The second function to explore is `names( )`:

```
> names(MMstat)
 [1] "ID"          "Age"          "Male"         "Weight"
 [5] "Height"      "Diabetes"     "COPD"         "LVEF"
 [9] "Creatinine"  "Aspirin"      "Broccoli"     "CPB"
[13] "CC"          "LOS"          "Mortality"    "Bleeding"
[17] "FUmortality" "FUtime"
```

This function returns the names of the variables in a dataset. Outlined above are the columns as they are entered in the example dataset, from column to 1 to 18 (i.e. the variable "`ID`" is located in column 1 and "`FUmortality`" and "`FUtime`" in columns 17 and 18, respectively).

The function `ls( )` returns the names of the variables in alphabetical order:

```
> ls(MMstat) #list alphabetic order
 [1] "Age"         "Aspirin"      "Bleeding"     "Broccoli"
 [5] "CC"          "COPD"         "CPB"          "Creatinine"
 [9] "Diabetes"    "FUmortality"  "FUtime"       "Height"
[13] "ID"          "LOS"          "LVEF"         "Male"
[17] "Mortality"   "Weight"
```

The head and tail of a dataset can be visualised with the function `head( )` and `tail( )` and they both return the first and last six rows of a dataset, respectively.

However, the most vital function is `str( )` (Fig. 3.4).

```
> str(MMstat)
```

As you can see, it returns at a glance the internal structure of a dataset (i.e. number of observations, classes of observations and also the levels (if any)). This is explained deeper in Chap. 4, where we discuss types of variables and how to convert them (e.g. from numeric to non-numeric). You might already notice above that some of the variables are miscoded. For example, in the "`Male`" variable, a subject's gender is identified by either 1 or 0, which leads "R" to code it as a numeric variable. This function may also tell us about any missing values.

The table below summarises some useful functions in "R" for data exploration:

```
> str(MMstat)
'data.frame':   500 obs. of  18 variables:
 $ ID         : int  107 224 155 494 48 486 194 140 333 282 ...
 $ Age        : int  19 22 86 85 83 23 27 83 83 30 ...
 $ Male       : int  0 1 1 0 0 0 0 1 0 0 ...
 $ Weight     : int  62 86 70 84 45 50 89 70 48 56 ...
 $ Height     : int  165 190 170 175 165 165 180 163 158 160 ...
 $ Diabetes   : int  0 0 1 0 0 0 0 0 0 0 ...
 $ COPD       : chr  "0" "0" "0" "0" ...
 $ LVEF       : int  60 53 65 71 54 55 60 51 54 55 ...
 $ Creatinine : num  0.53 0.84 0.89 1.44 0.91 0.5 1.23 0.81 0.67 0.64 ...
 $ Aspirin    : int  1 0 1 1 0 0 1 0 1 0 ...
 $ Broccoli   : chr  "y" "y" "n" "n" ...
 $ CPB        : int  61 93 123 50 40 89 93 50 72 52 ...
 $ CC         : int  39 49 94 30 29 37 66 20 38 30 ...
 $ LOS        : int  45 NA NA NA NA NA NA 5 NA NA ...
 $ Mortality  : int  0 0 0 0 0 0 0 0 0 0 ...
 $ Bleeding   : int  527 540 890 381 245 600 550 257 655 401 ...
 $ FUmortality: int  0 0 1 1 1 0 0 1 1 0 ...
 $ FUtime     : int  12 13 8 10 15 11 23 18 2 21 ...
```

Fig. 3.4 The function str( ) returns the nature of the variables (i.e. integer, characters) for the example dataset

Useful functions for dataset exploration	
`dim( )`	Outlines a dataset's dimensions (i.e. number of rows and columns)
`names( )`	Lists the names of the variables of a dataset in order of columns
`ls( )`	Lists the names of the variables of a dataset in alphabetical order
`head( )`	Lists the first six variables in a dataset
`tail( )`	Lists the last six variables in a dataset
`str( )`	Sets out the structure of a dataset, including the classes of the variables (i.e. numeric/non-numeric)

3.4 Subsetting

"R" allows different forms and possibilities for subsetting. By subsetting I refer to the possibility to obtain a "chunk" of the dataset (e.g. to extract only the data from individuals who include broccoli in their dietary intake before surgery). This can also be used for multiple subsetting (e.g. to extract the data of patients who include broccoli before surgery, who are male and who aged above 60 years old). This is very helpful. With only a few commands we can carry out a deep exploration of any dataset for descriptive analysis.

In order to perform subsetting, we use the operator `[]`.

We can start by creating two separate subsets. The first subset contains all the data of the individuals who include broccoli before surgery; the second contains all the data of those who do not include broccoli before surgery.

To perform subsetting in "R" we can use the basic built-in function (basic subsetting) in base-R, or for more advanced subsetting, we can use the `dplyr` package from the R-package `tidyverse`.

3.5 Subsetting with Base-R

Basic subsetting is described here. It is repeated later in this book.

One of the first things we may like to do is create two objects. One that contains all data about the broccoli group, and another that contains all data about the control (noBroccoli) group.

Here it is important to remember our research question. What are the effects (if any) of a broccoli dietary regimen on post-operative outcomes? Understanding the characteristics of each group is very important.

We use the following codes:

```
> broccoli<-MMstat[MMstat$Broccoli=='y',]
> nobroccoli<-MMstat[MMstat$Broccoli=='n',]
```

With the help of Fig. 3.5, further below I break down the code to help you better understand it layer by layer:

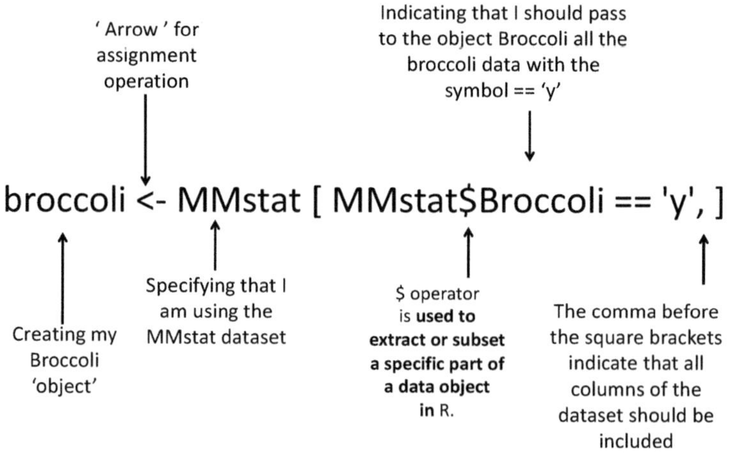

Fig. 3.5 Creating the object "broccoli"

In the first line code, to the new object `Broccoli` we assign `<-` all the information contained in the dataset `MMstat` that relates to patients who include the broccoli dietary regimen before surgery `Broccoli=='y'`. The operator `[ ]` is crucial for subsetting. It comes after the dataset of interest and specifies which variables to subset from the dataset. In our case we are interested in subsetting the variable `Broccoli`. Note, `Broccoli` is a nominal variable that has two coded levels "`y`" and "`n`". Once again "R" is very meticulous. If you pay attention, in the dataset the variable is coded as `Broccoli` with a capital B, and any misspelling will return an error.

What is the meaning of the `$` (dollar sign) operator? This dollar sign is one of the most common operators in "R". In the examples above, it simply tells "R" to retrieve from the dataset `MMstat` the variable `Broccoli`. If we were to simply type `MMstat$Broccoli`, "R" would return all the information about the variable `Broccoli`.

What is the meaning of the -- operator? It is a Boolean operator, meaning there are two possible values (in this case, true or false). The example above, which creates the `broccoli` object, tells "R" to consider only the `Broccoli=='y'` participants. That way only the patients who included the broccoli dietary regimen before surgery will be included in the `broccoli` object. Finally, at the end there is a comma`,` in the code. A comma here is to specify which columns of the dataset are to be included. In this example, by not entering any numbers after the comma command, it tells "R" to select *all* the columns in the dataset for `Broccoli=='y'` subjects. If a number was entered after the comma (e.g. "...`Broccoli=='y',1]`"), "R" would only retrieve data from column 1.

The table below summarises common operators in "R":

Common operators in "R"	
?	This is the help operator. It is used in combination with a function, (e.g. `?mean`) and displays the help menu in the lower right pane of the four-pane workspace of "R"
<-	This assigns the value to the right of it, to the object at the left of it (e.g. `broccoli<-MMstat`, where `MMstat` is assigned to the `broccoli` object)
$	This is one of the most common operators in "R". It tells "R" to retrieve a specific variable from a certain dataset (e.g. `MMstat$Broccoli` tells "R" to extract the variable `Broccoli` from the dataset `MMstat`)
' '	Any information in between single quotation marks will be transformed as literal and "R" will search only for that exact character or sequence of characters
#	This is used for commenting; it tells "R" to ignore all characters after the # and to move on to the next line; it does not affect the capability of "R" to run the next line
`c()`	The "c" stands for concatenate, it will combine the contents of the brackets (numeric and non-numeric) into a vector
+	This is also a form of concatenation and is used in writing long scripts with multiple lines, rather than "R" interpreting each new line as a new command; it scans it all as one single command

==	A Boolean operator is used to collate data when there is one of two possible values to be retrieved, usually true or false (e.g. `MMstat$Broccoli=='y'` collates all "true" `Broccoli` data from `MMstat` (i.e. it collates specified information from all patients who include the broccoli dietary regimen pre-surgery))

With the codes below, we split the dataset `MMstat` into two separate groups:

```
> broccoli<-MMstat[MMstat$Broccoli=='y',]
> nobroccoli<-MMstat[MMstat$Broccoli=='n',]
```

The first group, `broccoli`, contains all the information about subjects who include the broccoli dietary regimen before surgery. The second group, `nobroccoli`, contains all the information about subjects who do not.

What is the value of having two separated groups/vectors? The process of subsetting helps with both exploratory and descriptive analyses, as well as inferential statistics. Let us assume we want to explore differences (if any) based on the mean age between the two groups `broccoli` and `nobroccoli`. We simply use the `summary( )` function:

```
> summary(broccoli$Age)
   Min. 1st Qu.  Median    Mean 3rd Qu.    Max.
  19.00   57.50   66.00   63.83   72.50   86.00
> summary(nobroccoli$Age)
   Min. 1st Qu.  Median    Mean 3rd Qu.    Max.
  14.00   54.00   65.00   62.82   73.00   86.00
```

Here, the `summary( )` function tells us that the average age of the two groups is similar.

Now, since we have carried out subsetting we can put the numbers into graphics (Fig. 3.6):

```
> boxplot(broccoli$Age, nobroccoli$Age,col=c('red', 'blue'),
xaxt='n', main='Age y/o in the two groups')
> axis(1, at=1:2, labels=c('Broccoli','noBroccoli'))
```

Again, using this visual representation with `boxplot`, it is possible to see the median (the black lines inside the boxplot) is similar between the two groups, with some variability differences between the groups, and more outliers in the Broccoli group. This book explains `boxplot`, as well as hypothesis testing, in more detail eventually. In fact, to understand better if the average differs, we should select the appropriate test according to normality distribution and other assumptions. But here, our focus is only on subsetting coding.

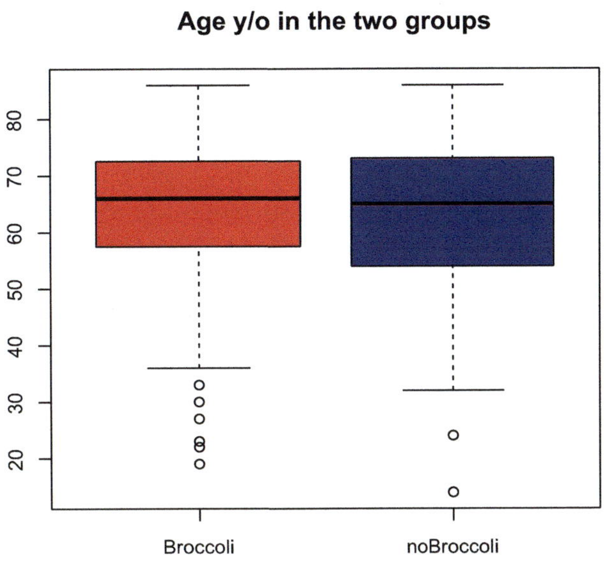

Fig. 3.6 Boxplot of Broccoli vs noBroccoli groups

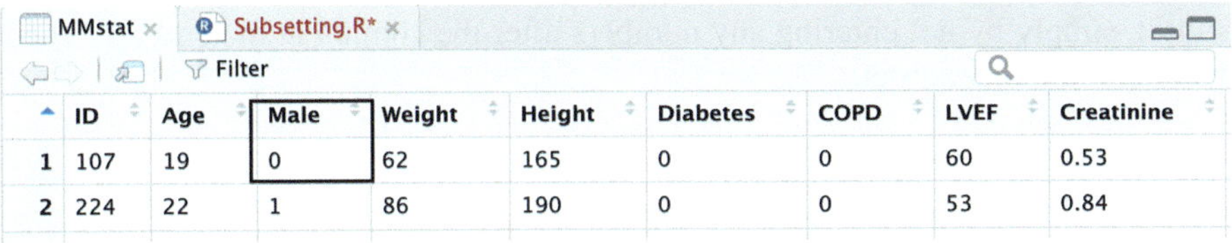

	ID	Age	Male	Weight	Height	Diabetes	COPD	LVEF	Creatinine
1	107	19	0	62	165	0	0	60	0.53
2	224	22	1	86	190	0	0	53	0.84

Fig. 3.7 Subsetting: identifying the first row (n=1) and the third column (n=3)

3.6 More Examples of Basic Subsetting

With the built-in function in "R", square bracket `[ , ]` is the operator for subsetting. This command indicates what data to select from a given dataset. You will see there is also a comma inserted inside the brackets `[ , ]`. Numbers to the left of the comma indicate the row(s), while numbers to the right indicate the column(s) (Fig. 3.7):

```
> MMstat[1,3]
[1] 0
```

Figure 3.7 shows the 0 returned by "R" is the value from the dataset which corresponds to the coordinates given in the code, i.e. *first* row and *third* column `[1,3]` of the dataset `MMstat`.

Let's carry out a more interesting subsetting code. Perhaps we want to know how many individuals over 50 years old are included in the dataset `MMstat`.

```
> Ageover50<-MMstat$Age[MMstat$Age>50]
> length(Ageover50)
[1] 421
```

To do so, first we create a new object named `Ageover50` and assign `<-` to it the `Age` variable from the `MMstat` dataset `MMstat$Age`, further specifying to only include values greater than 50 `[MMstat$Age>50]`. Next, we use the `length` function to know how many individuals are contained in the new `Ageover50` object.

Furthermore, perhaps we are interested in obtaining a dataset of patients over or equal to 50 years old. To do so, we must subset *the entire* `MMstat` dataset rather than just the column `MMstat$Age` and tell "R" that all columns should be included by not entering any numbers after the comma, as set out in the code below:

```
> Ageover50<-MMstat[MMstat$Age>=50,]
> View(Ageover50)
```

As you can see, first we subset the entire dataset `MMstat` and prompt "R" to include all patients with an `Age` greater than or equal to 50 years old `>=50`, as well as to return all information from the entire dataset related to the patients in this new subset, simply by not entering any numbers after the comma at the end `,]`. Then, we `View` the new subset:

```
View(Ageover50)
```

Let us probe further and introduce the `&` operator. Perhaps we are interested, as part of the exploratory analysis, to produce a subset that contains only patients older than 50 years old, who include the broccoli dietary regimen before surgery and who are *also* taking aspirin.

```
> Ageover50<-MMstat[MMstat$Age>50 & MMstat$Broccoli=='y' &
MMstat$Aspirin=='1',]
> View(Ageover50)
```

The vector has still the same name `Ageover50`, but now contains only patients with an `Age` greater than 50 `MMstat$Age>50`, who include the broccoli dietary regimen before surgery `MMstat$Broccoli=='y'` and are taking aspirin `MMstat$Aspirin=='1'`.

Now we are at this stage, let's plot the average age of the Broccoli individuals who are over or equal to 50 years old and who are also taking aspirin against the same counterparts of the noBroccoli group. First, we use the following codes:

```
> Ageover50broccoli<-MMstat[MMstat$Age>=50 & MMstat$Broccoli=='y'
& MMstat$Aspirin=='1',]
>Ageover50nobroccoli<-MMstat[MMstat$Age>=50 & MMstat$Broccoli=='n'
& MMstat$Aspirin=='1',]
```

With this, two new vectors are created. The `Ageover50broccoli` vector contains patients greater than or equal to 50 years old `MMstat$Age>=50`, who are including the broccoli dietary regimen before surgery `MMstat$Broccoli=='y'` and are also taking aspirin `MMstat$Aspirin=='1'`. The `Ageover50nobroccoli` vector contains patients who are also greater than or equal to 50 years old `MMstat$Age>=50`, but who aren't including the broccoli dietary regimen before surgery `MMstat$Broccoli=='n'`; however, they too are taking aspirin `MMstat$Aspirin=='1'`.

Now, to visualise the age of these two groups using `boxplot` (Fig. 3.8):

```
> boxplot(Ageover50broccoli$Age, Ageover50nobroccoli$Age,
col=c('red', 'blue'), boxwex=0.4, ylim=c(50,100), ylab='years
old', main= 'Patients over 50 with Aspirin')
> axis(1, at=1:2, labels=c('Broccoli','noBroccoli'))
```

Note that so far we have only produced plots using basic functions in "R" and they do look quite basic. We discuss further in the book which statistical test to use for hypothesis testing.

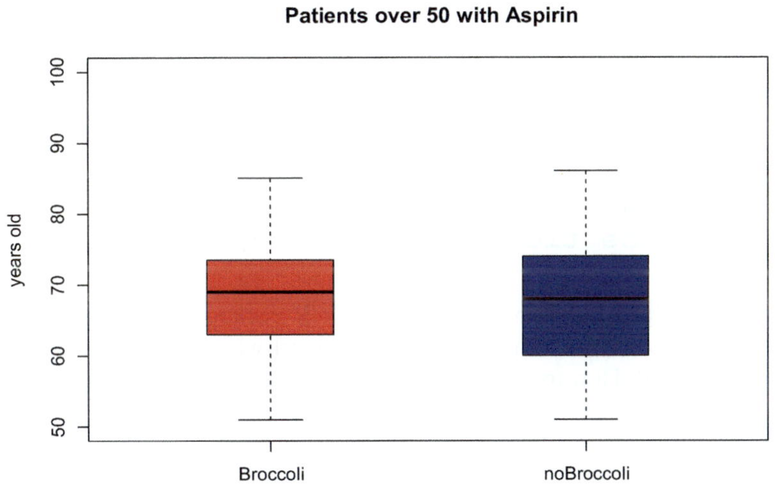

Fig. 3.8 Boxplot of Broccoli vs noBroccoli patients who are 50 years old and over and who are taking aspirin

Next, let's say we are interested in looking at only the patients who include the broccoli dietary regimen and who are within a certain age range (i.e. patients between 80 and 85 years old). We can use the code below:

```
> broccoli<-MMstat[MMstat$Broccoli=='y' & MMstat$Age>='80' & MMstat$Age<='85',]
```

Note that this latest code includes specifications both for age greater than or equal to 80 `>='80'` *and* age less than or equal to 85 `<='85'`.

There is a script named `EDA.R` which can be downloaded from GitHub and which shows other examples of subsetting for you to practice.

3.7 The Attach Function

The operator `$` extracts a certain variable from a certain dataset, e.g. `MMstat$Age` when extracting age data from the example dataset. When working with a longer code, instead of typing the name of a dataset every time, we can attach it just once using the `attach` function:

```
> mean(MMstat$Age)
[1] 63.23
> attach(MMstat)# by attaching the dataset MMstat I do not need to
retype the name of the dataset again
> mean(Age)
[1] 63.23
```

"R" will continue to extract from the attached dataset for all further lines of code, until commanded otherwise.

3.8 Storing a Dataset as a Tibble for Use with the tidyverse R-Package

In order to use `dplyr` (part of the `tidyverse` R-package) as a subsetting tool, we must first store a dataset as a tibble (a local dataset which is ultimately neater and less cumbersome). How to do this is set out below, using the example dataset:

```
> mmsubset<-as_tibble(MMstat)
```

So far, we have covered some useful functions and operators for subsetting; however, an even more in-depth and detailed description of subsetting, including using `dplyr` within `tidyverse`, can be found in the script named `Chapter 3.EDA.R` at the following GitHub link:

https://github.com/mmlondon77/Biobook.git.

3.9 Frequently Used Subsetting Functions

Outlined in this section are some of the most used functions for subsetting in "R":

1. `filter( )`

   This function filters by row. Let us create a dataset chunk called `broccolidpl` which contains only `Broccoli== 'y'` subjects:

```
> broccolidpl<-filter(mmsubset, Broccoli=='y')
```

Filtering is very easy and intuitive. Next, we can create a subset of patients including broccoli `Broccoli== 'y'`, but without COPD `COPD== '0'`, or of individuals greater than or equal to 80 years old `Age>='80'`:

```
> broccolidpl<-filter(mmsubset, Broccoli=='y', COPD=='0')
> broccolidpl<-filter(mmsubset, Age>='80')
```

Then when we have a variable with more than two levels (e.g. `Diabetes`), we can use the index operator `%in%` or the pipe operator `|`:

```
> broccolidpl<-filter(mmsubset, Diabetes %in% c('1', '2'))#select-
ing all patients with Diabetes value 1 or 2
> broccolidpl<-filter(mmsubset, Diabetes=='1'| Diabetes=='0')#
selecting all patients with Diabetes value 1 or 0
```

Remember the function `view( )` to visualise the file after subsetting, e.g.:

```
> view(broccolidpl)
```

which returns the function table including only those subjects with one of two levels of the covariate "Diabetes" after subsetting (Fig. 3.9):

	ID	Age	Male	Weight	Height	Diabetes	COPD	LVEF	Creatinine	Aspirin
1	107	19	0	62	165	0	0	60	0.53	1
2	224	22	1	86	190	0	0	53	0.84	0
3	155	86	1	70	170	1	0	65	0.89	1
4	494	85	0	84	175	0	0	71	1.44	1
5	48	83	0	45	165	0	0	54	0.91	0

Fig. 3.9 Viewing subsetting using the filter function. Selecting (filtering by row) patients with diabetes levels 0 and 1 (Diabetes has three levels). The table ( ) function which follows also confirms we excluded the third level 2

2. `select( )`

   This function filters by column. Let us select the columns with `Diabetes` and `Broccoli`.

```
> broccolidpl<-dplyr::select(mmsubset, Diabetes, Broccoli)# Note that with the symbol :: I specify that the function select comes from the package dplyr
> broccolidpl<-dplyr::select(mmsubset, ID:Broccoli)# Selecting columns from ID to Broccoli only
> broccolidpl<-dplyr::select(mmsubset,starts_with('Bro'))# Selecting only columns that start with 'Bro'
```

3. `filter( )` *and* `select( )`

   It is often necessary to combine the functions `filter( )` and `select( )` (this is known as chaining). Let's make an example. Say we are interested in selecting only columns `Broccoli` and `Age` and including only the patients above 80 years old (Fig. 3.10):

```
> broccolidpl<-filter(dplyr::select(mmsubset, Broccoli, Age), Age > 80)#chaining select and filter
> head(broccolidpl)# the function "head" returns the first 6 observations
```

   This is similar to:

```
> broccolidpl<-mmsubset %>%
  dplyr::select(Broccoli, Age)%>%
  filter(Age>80)
```

   Note that the `%>%` operator sends the `select` function to the `mmsubset` tibble, prompting to select the columns `Broccoli` and `Age` and filtering for `Age>80`.

```
> head(broccolidpl)
# A tibble: 6 × 2
  Broccoli   Age
  <chr>    <int>
1 n           86
2 n           85
3 n           83
4 n           83
5 n           83
6 n           83
```

Fig. 3.10 Applying both filter and select, subsetting for two columns (Broccoli and Age) including only the rows with age above 80 years old

4. `arrange( )`

This function re-orders the rows. For example, we want to `select( )` for `Broccoli` and `Age` but this time to arrange `Age` in ascending order (Fig. 3.11):

```
> broccolidpl<-mmsubset %>%
  dplyr::select(Broccoli, Age)%>%
  arrange(asc=Age)
> View(broccolidpl)
```

5. `mutate( )`

With the `mutate( )` function we can add new columns with new variables into a dataset. In cardiac surgery we have a surgical period where the patient is connected to the heart-lung machine and this is coded as `CPB` (cardio-pulmonary bypass time).

There is also a surgical period where the heart is connected to the heart-lung machine but also stands still to allow surgeons to operate comfortably and this is coded as `CC` (cross-clamp or ischaemic time).

The example below shows how to add a column which contains variables of the difference between `CPB` and `CC`, and this will be named `ONBH` (i.e. on pump beating heart) (Fig. 3.12).

Fig. 3.11 Viewing results of arrange function which allows us to order a variable in level, ascending or descending order

	Broccoli	Age
1	n	14
2	y	19
3	y	22
4	y	23
5	n	24
6	n	24
7	y	27
8	y	30
9	y	30
10	n	32

Fig. 3.12 Viewing the new column ONBH added with the mutate function

	Broccoli	Age	CC	CPB	ONBH
1	y	19	39	61	22
2	y	22	49	93	44
3	n	86	94	123	29
4	n	85	30	50	20
5	n	83	29	40	11
6	y	23	37	89	52
7	y	27	66	93	27

```
> broccolidpl<-mmsubset %>%
  dplyr::select(Broccoli, Age, CC, CPB)%>%
  mutate(ONBH=CPB-CC)
> View(broccolidpl)
```

6. `summarise( )`

   This function is very helpful since it reduces variables to values. Let's make an example. Say we are interested, at a glance, on the average bleeding in the `Broccoli=='y'` vs `Broccoli=='n'` groups. In this case, we first use the `group_by( )` function and follow up with the `summarise( )` function:

```
> broccolidpl<-mmsubset %>%
  group_by(Broccoli)%>%
  summarise(Averagebleeding=mean(Bleeding, na.rm=T))
> View(broccolidpl)
```

   Note that we first use the `group_by( )` function to obtain the two groups `Broccoli=='y'` vs `Broccoli=='n'`. Then by using the `summarise( )` function we create the `Averagebleeding` object that contains the `mean` of `Bleeding`. Finally, in case of missing values we prompt "R" to remove them with the `na.rm=T` function (Fig. 3.13).

   Or if we'd rather see the standard deviation, instead of the mean:

```
> broccolidpl<-mmsubset %>%
  group_by(Broccoli)%>%
   summarise(Averagebleeding=sd(Bleeding, na.rm=T))#We have
specified to calculate the standard deviation instead of the mean.
```

7. `summarise_each( )`

   We can use the `summarise_each( )` function after another function. The following examples demonstrate first using the `group_by` function for the continuous `Age` variable, then using `summarise_each( )` to find out, according to age, the average `Bleeding` and `CPB` time or the `min` and `max` values for `Bleeding`:

Fig. 3.13 Viewing the result from the summarise function

Filter

	Broccoli	Avaragebleeding
1	n	581.7003
2	y	475.3793

```
> broccolidpl<-mmsubset %>%
  group_by(Age)%>%
  summarise_each(mean, Bleeding, CPB)

> broccolidpl<-mmsubset %>%
  group_by(Age)%>%
 summarise_each(funs(min(.,na.rm=TRUE), max(., na.rm=TRUE)),
matches('Bleeding'))
```

8. `tally( )`
   It is also possible to use the function `tally( )` to count observations according to a specific strata (Fig. 3.14):

```
> broccolidpl<-mmsubset %>%
  group_by(Age, Broccoli)%>%
  tally(sort=TRUE)
> View(broccolidpl)
```

Subsetting can be considered a part of EDA. It may be carried out with basic functions in "R" or with more advanced methods provided by `dplyr` within `tidyverse`. Although the latter may seem more complex, it requires shorter code than the basic function. Other examples for you to practice are given in the related script called `Chapter 3.EDA.R` which accompanies this chapter.

Fig. 3.14 Viewing the result of the tally function to count the observations according to strata. The first row tells we have n=13 individuals in the no Broccoli group of age 51 years old, row 2 tells we have 13 patients in the Broccoli group of 72 years old, etc

	Age	Broccoli	n
1	51	n	13
2	72	y	13
3	71	n	12
4	74	n	12
5	75	n	12
6	59	y	11
7	61	n	11
8	66	n	10
9	70	n	10
10	71	y	10
11	59	n	9
12	63	n	9
13	67	n	9

3.10 Conclusions

Exploratory data analysis (EDA) is used to manipulate data within datasets to summarise certain characteristics. EDA leads to a better understanding of data, identification of potential data patterns and magnitude and nature of any missing data. It also helps to formulate an original research question. Data partitioning and subsetting is part of EDA and can be carried out with built-in functions in "R" or with other tools such as `dplyr`, part of the `tidyverse` R-package. This chapter demonstrates how to perform subsetting and introduces the creation of simple plots.

Further Readings

Brendan RE. Introduction to R – tidyverse. https://bookdown.org/ansellbr/WEHI_tidyR_course_book/

Irizarry RA. Introduction to data science: data analysis and prediction algorithms with R. CRC Press; 2019.

Pearson RK. Exploratory data analysis using R. Morrisville: CRC Press; 2018.

Peng, R. (2012). Exploratory data analysis with R. Morrisville. Available from: Lulu.com

Wicham H, Grolemund G. R for data science. Available from: https://r4ds.had.co.nz/exploratory-data-analysis.html

Chapter 4
Data Types in "R"

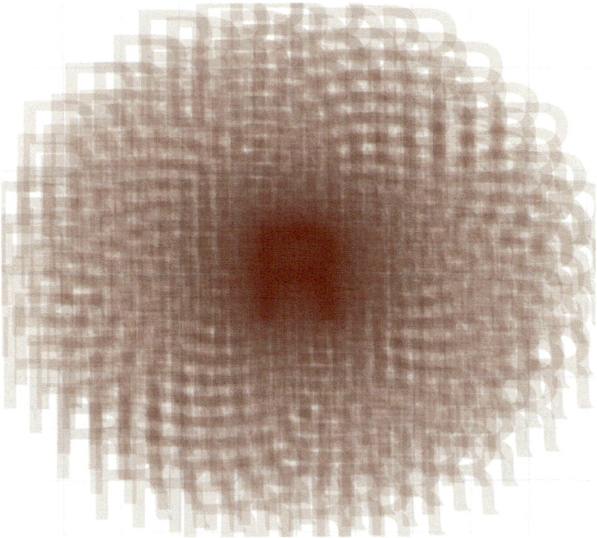

4.1 Software and R-Packages Required for This Chapter

If you haven't already, you need to download and install base-R and R-studio as set out in Chap. 2 under the heading "Downloading "R" and R-studio".

The relevant R-packages needed for this chapter are:

- Amelia—it can be downloaded at:
  https://gking.harvard.edu/amelia

M. Moscarelli, *Biostatistics With 'R': A Guide for Medical Doctors*,
https://doi.org/10.1007/978-3-031-33073-5_4

- tableone—it can be downloaded at:
  https://github.com/kaz-yos/tableone

4.2 Where to Find the Example Dataset and the Script for This Chapter

If you haven't already downloaded the supplementary dataset named `MMstat.csv` created as a practical example for use throughout this book, you will find it at the link that follows. The script for this chapter named `Chapter 4.Data types.R` can also be found and downloaded at the following link:

https://github.com/mmlondon77/Biobook.git

4.3 What Is the Nature of Our Data?

The example dataset `MMstat` has many columns; each column identifies a different variable, e.g. `Male` is coded with either `1` or `0` (`1` being male, `0` being female), `Age` contains the age of each patient, and `Creatinine` outlines each patient's blood creatinine level expressed in mg/dl, etc. `Male` is non-numeric, even though it is coded with numbers. Both `Age` and `Creatinine` are numeric, yet `Age` does not contain decimals, whereas `Creatinine` does. There is also `Broccoli`, entered as `y` or `n`, which is therefore non-numeric.

What is the difference between `Age` and `Creatinine`? Shall we consider them both as numeric data? What is the structure of the `Male` and `Broccoli` variables?

Before delving into the nature of our data, I should clarify that "R" broadly recognises two kinds of data:

a) Numeric (quantitative)
b) Non-numeric (qualitative)

4.4 Numeric Data

The `Creatinine` variable is numeric. It contains numbers with decimals. All variables containing numbers are considered numeric.

Let's use "R" to check the structure of the variable. To do so, we use one of two functions, `str( )` or `class( )`:

```
> str(MMstat$Creatinine)
 num [1:500] 0.53 0.84 0.89 1.44 0.91 0.5 1.23 0.81 0.67 0.64 ...
> class(MMstat$Creatinine)
[1] "numeric"
```

"R" shows that the `Creatinine` variable contains numeric data, from 1 to 500, and sets out that the numeric values contain decimals.

4.5 Integer

If a numeric variable does not contain decimals, "R" will recognise it as an integer, e.g. `Age` is usually entered in years without decimals. Other examples include the number of children in a family, the number of coronary artery bypass surgeries that may have been performed for each patient or the number of coronary stents each patient may have. Those are units that do not contain decimals. Let's check the structure or class of the `Age` variable:

```
> str(MMstat$Age)
 int [1:500] 19 22 86 85 83 23 27 83 83 30 ...
> class(MMstat$Age)
[1] "integer"
```

This shows that the `Age` column has 500 observations; it does not contain decimals and is an integer. This is fair since a discrete numeric variable (i.e. without decimals) should be identified as an integer.

There can only be a discrete number of coronary artery bypass grafts performed, from 0 to say a maximum of 5 or 6. The range is limited, but most importantly you cannot perform 1.5 bypasses nor 2.5 coronary stent surgeries. These variables will never have decimals!

4.6 Character

Any data containing text can be classified as a character, e.g. `Broccoli` data is stored as `y` or `n`, with `y` identifying patients who are including the broccoli dietary regimen before surgery and `n` identifying those who are not.

```
> str(MMstat$Broccoli)
 chr [1:500] "y" "y" "n" "n" "n" "y" "y" "n" "n" "y" "n" "n" "n" ...
 > class(MMstat$Broccoli)
[1] "character"
```

"R" confirms that `Broccoli` is classed as a character. Note that any data, which appears in "R" between single or double speech marks (e.g. the `"y"` and `"n"` data above), will be considered a character, no matter if it contains characters or not.

```
> x<-c('1', '2', '3')
> class(x)
[1] "character"
```

Similarly, the object `x` is created and contains numbers 1–3. Since those numbers are entered between single speech marks this time, "R" also classifies `x` as a character.

4.7 Factors

Factors are a special kind of character data, they are stored as text but have few non-hierarchical levels, e.g. gender (male and female). But what about the variable `Broccoli`? Is it not the same as gender? From the point of view of "R", both factors and characters are identical. `Broccoli` is a character as well as a factor.

To clarify, variables with many possibilities can be stored as a *character*; variables with only two non-hierarchical values can be stored as a *factor*. Either way, "R" will recognise them as non-numeric. Factors can also be named as categorical variables.

If we create an object called `therapy`, which contains the possibilities of treatments for coronary artery disease, we can ask "R" how many possibilities the `therapy` object has by using the `levels( )` function:

```
> therapy <- factor(c("no", "surgery", "stent", 'no', 'surgery',
'surgery'))
> levels(therapy)
[1] "no"      "stent"   "surgery"
```

The `therapy` variable contains three possibilities or levels. It is certainly a character and also broadly speaking it is non-numeric.

4.8 Variable Classification

As outlined earlier, "R" assumes we deal with two main classes of data, numeric and non-numeric. Numeric represents both continuous values (e.g. values with decimals such as blood creatinine levels) and integer, for discrete values (e.g. values which are counted and therefore without decimals such as age and the number of stents which have been implanted in each patient (if any)). All non-numeric variables are characters (containing two or more levels) or also factors if they contain only two levels (e.g. the male variable which identifies the gender of each patient).

Numeric variables can also be defined as *quantitative*, since they are expressed in numbers, while non-numeric also as *qualitative*, since they represent characteristics. The last classification that is important to understand with regard to qualitative variables is the distinction between nominal and ordinal.

Nominal values can be factors and/or characters (e.g. eye colour, gender) whereby all levels are equal, i.e. one eye colour is no more important than another and female gender is equal to male gender.

Ordinal variables can only be characters; they have *hierarchical levels*, e.g. the diabetes variable has three levels: no diabetes, non-insulin-dependent diabetes and insulin-dependent diabetes mellitus, where some conditions are more consequential than others. Another example of a non-numeric, qualitative, ordinal variable is the NYHA (New York Heart Association) class for dyspnoea. It ranges from I to IV, whereby I is characterised as no limitation and IV dyspnoea at rest. Obviously, NYHA class IV is much worse than other levels. Similarly, the Canadian Cardiovascular Society grading of angina is also considered a non-numeric, qualitative, ordinal variable.

The tree diagram below summarises at a glance the variables classification (Fig. 4.1):

Data type	Example
Numeric (continuous) (quantitative variable)	Creatinine (e.g. 1.3 mg/dl) numbers with decimals
Integer (discrete) (quantitative variable)	Age (e.g. 34 y/o) numbers without decimals

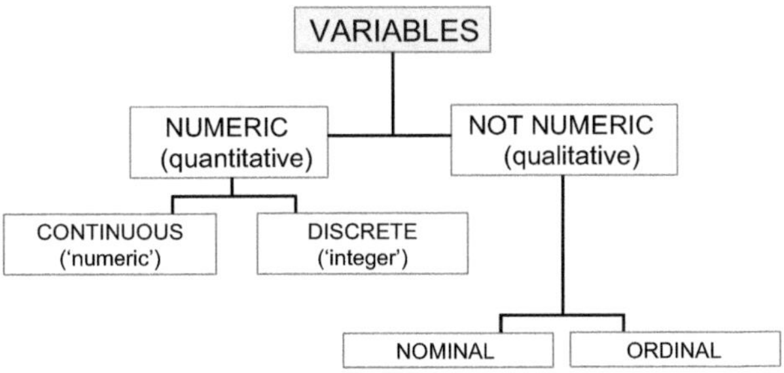

Fig. 4.1 Tree diagram setting out data types and classifications

Data type	Example
Factor (qualitative variable)	Gender, two non-hierarchical levels (male/female)
Character nominal (qualitative variable with no hierarchical order)	Eye colour, many levels
Character ordinal (qualitative variable with hierarchical order)	NYHA class for dyspnoea that goes from I to IV (none to worst symptoms)

4.9 Misleading Data Encoding

We might note that we have some erroneous or misleading data encoded in our dataset `MMstat`. But first, let us check the structure and class of our dataset. This is a very important part of the tidying up process of statistical analysis. We use the function `str( )` again (Fig. 4.2):

```
> str(MMstat)
```

We can now visualise the class and structure of all 18 variables in our example dataset. This is mandatory before any further analysis. As aforementioned, we can note some misleading data encoded in the dataset `MMstat`, e.g. `Male` is coded with

```
> str(MMstat)
'data.frame':   500 obs. of  18 variables:
 $ ID         : int  107 224 155 494 48 486 194 140 333 282 ...
 $ Age        : int  19 22 86 85 83 23 27 83 83 30 ...
 $ Male       : int  0 1 1 0 0 0 0 1 0 0 ...
 $ Weight     : int  62 86 70 84 45 50 89 70 48 56 ...
 $ Height     : int  165 190 170 175 165 165 180 163 158 160 ...
 $ Diabetes   : int  0 0 1 0 0 0 0 0 0 0 ...
 $ COPD       : int  0 0 0 0 0 0 0 0 0 0 ...
 $ LVEF       : int  60 53 65 71 54 55 60 51 54 55 ...
 $ Creatinine : num  0.53 0.84 0.89 1.44 0.91 0.5 1.23 0.81 0.67 0.64 ...
 $ Aspirin    : int  1 0 1 1 0 0 1 0 1 0 ...
 $ Broccoli   : chr  "y" "y" "n" "n" ...
 $ CPB        : int  61 93 123 50 40 89 93 50 72 52 ...
 $ CC         : int  39 49 94 30 29 37 66 20 38 30 ...
 $ LOS        : int  45 NA NA NA NA NA NA 5 NA NA ...
 $ Mortality  : int  0 0 0 0 0 0 0 0 0 0 ...
 $ Bleeding   : int  527 540 890 381 245 600 550 257 655 401 ...
 $ FUmortality: int  0 0 1 1 1 0 0 1 1 0 ...
 $ FUtime     : int  12 13 8 10 15 11 23 18 2 21 ...
```

Fig. 4.2 Visualising data structure with the str( ) function

1 or 0, so "R" returns it as a numeric variable (an integer). Yet it is in fact non-numeric (qualitative), and because it has two levels, it is also a factor.

Similarly with Diabetes, COPD, Aspirin, Mortality and FUmortality, again, these variables are defined by "R" as integers, yet they are in fact non-numeric (qualitative). However, Diabetes also has three hierarchical levels (no diabetes, non-insulin dependent and insulin dependent), so it should be defined as an ordinal variable. All others COPD, Aspirin, Mortality and FUmortality, like Male, are also factors. We can ignore the variable ID (first column). It is not relevant for the analysis and only represents the anonymous ID of each patient. We need to assign the exact class to each variable before any other further action. To do so, we can use the commands below:

```
> varsToFactor <- c("Male", "Mortality","Aspirin", "COPD",
"FUmortality")
> MMstat[varsToFactor] <- lapply(MMstat[varsToFactor], factor)
```

Basically, we create a new object that contains all the variables that we need to convert to factor variables varsToFactor. Then we reshape the MMstat dataset to attach the new modified variables. To do so, we use the function lapply.

Next, in the same way, we re-assign the class for the diabetes variable:

Let us re-check the class and structure of the dataset MMstat after variable transformation (Fig. 4.3):

We have now successfully converted the structure of "Male", "COPD", "Aspirin", "Mortality" and "FUmortality" from numeric integers to non-numeric factors and "Diabetes" to a non-numeric, ordinal character.

```
> str(MMstat)
'data.frame':   500 obs. of  18 variables:
 $ ID         : int  107 224 155 494 48 486 194 140 333 282 ...
 $ Age        : int  19 22 86 85 83 23 27 83 83 30 ...
 $ Male       : Factor w/ 2 levels "0","1": 1 2 2 1 1 1 1 2 1 1 ...
 $ Weight     : int  62 86 70 84 45 50 89 70 48 56 ...
 $ Height     : int  165 190 170 175 165 165 180 163 158 160 ...
 $ Diabetes   : Factor w/ 3 levels "0","1","2": 1 1 2 1 1 1 1 1 1 1 ...
 $ COPD       : Factor w/ 2 levels "0","1": 1 1 1 1 1 1 1 1 1 1 ...
 $ LVEF       : int  60 53 65 71 54 55 60 51 54 55 ...
 $ Creatinine : num  0.53 0.84 0.89 1.44 0.91 0.5 1.23 0.81 0.67 0.64 ...
 $ Aspirin    : Factor w/ 2 levels "0","1": 2 1 2 2 1 1 2 1 2 1 ...
 $ Broccoli   : chr  "y" "y" "n" "n" ...
 $ CPB        : int  61 93 123 50 40 89 93 50 72 52 ...
 $ CC         : int  39 49 94 30 29 37 66 20 38 30 ...
 $ LOS        : int  45 NA NA NA NA NA NA 5 NA NA ...
 $ Mortality  : Factor w/ 2 levels "0","1": 1 1 1 1 1 1 1 1 1 1 ...
 $ Bleeding   : int  527 540 890 381 245 600 550 257 655 401 ...
 $ FUmortality: Factor w/ 2 levels "0","1": 1 1 2 2 2 1 1 2 2 1 ...
 $ FUtime     : int  12 13 8 10 15 11 23 18 2 21 ...
```

Fig. 4.3 Data structure after manipulation

Note that the function `str( )` also outlines for us the number of levels there are within relevant variables.

The dataset also contains missing values. They are coded as `NA`. Missing values may heavily affect statistical analysis. Some of them can be left undisturbed, some others need to be removed, whereas some others need to be replaced.

4.10 Different Types of Variables Need Different Types of Statistical Analysis

We cannot compute the mean for non-numeric variables (e.g. patients with `COPD`). It also does not make sense to calculate the mode (the variables with highest frequency), as there would be few observations. Later in the book, we will investigate how correlation is carried out only for continuous numeric variables, chi-squared test for qualitative (non-numeric) variables and ANOVA for quantitative and qualitative variables.

This is why it is pivotal to understand the nature of the variables but also important to code them correctly. When data was entered into the fictitious dataset `MMstat`, the `Diabetes` variable was coded with numbers, from `0` to `2` outlining three levels (`0`=no diabetes, `1`=non-insulin-dependent diabetes, `2`=insulin-dependent diabetes). When the file is originally imported, “R” recognises the variable as numeric (integer) since the data contained within it is numbers without decimals. Theoretically, the mean could be computed, yet it would not make any logical sense. This is trickier when we have variables such as the number of coronary artery bypass grafts performed, e.g. some patients may have undergone anywhere from 1 to 5, or in some cases even 6, grafts, yet we cannot compute the average, since we cannot split a graft in two. This is also important when we perform regression analysis (as part of the inferential analysis), we must ensure beforehand that all variables are coded correctly.

4.11 Data Transformation and the Benefit of Continuous Variables

Theoretically, continuous variables convey more information than non-numeric ones. Let us assume that we want to test if including the broccoli dietary regimen has any effect in relation to age. We hypothesise that the older the patients, the more evident the benefits of broccoli are. To explore our hypothesis, we establish a conventional cut-off; let’s say 60 years old. In this case we transform the continuous variable `Age` into a factorial variable, being `0`= individual below 60 years old and `1`= equal to or above 60 years old. This is acceptable, and the subsetting can be performed as follows with the function `ifelse`:

Fig. 4.4 Creating the column "newage"

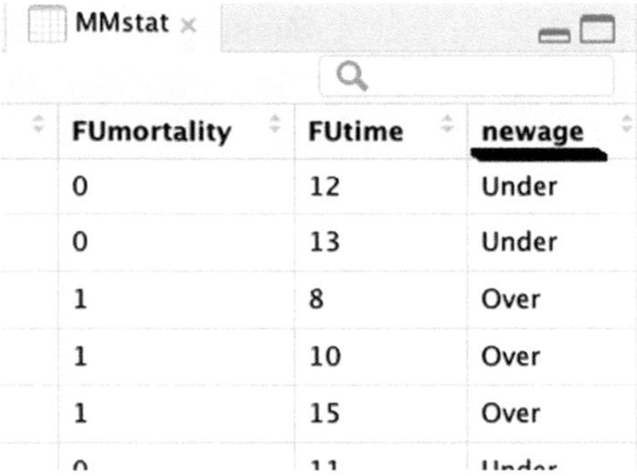

FUmortality	FUtime	newage
0	12	Under
0	13	Under
1	8	Over
1	10	Over
1	15	Over

```
> MMstat$newage<-ifelse(MMstat$Age>='60', yes='Over', no='Under')
```

From this, a new column `MMstat$newage` is created containing individuals aged >= 60 coded as `Over` and individuals not aged >= 60 coded as `Under`. This is added automatically to our dataset (Fig. 4.4).

While this is feasible, and commonly used in many scientific papers, we should keep the variables in the original form. This will become clearer when we explore regression analysis further in the book. Regression on binary outcome (i.e. over or under in this example) will return an odds ratio (binary logistic regression), whereas regression on continuous outcome will return a coefficient (slope). The latter is more informative, as we can make predictions from it.

4.12 Missing Values

How complete is our dataset `MMstat`? Often datasets contain missing observations, and our example dataset is no different. The quickest way to visualise the level of completeness of a dataset is to use the function `missmap` from the `Amelia` R-package (Fig. 4.5):

```
> install.packages('Amelia')
> library (Amelia)
> missmap(MMstat, y.at=500, col=c('red', 'green'), rank.order
= FALSE)
```

The package is named after the female aviator Amelia Earhart who went missing in 1937.

This `missmap` tells us that we have missing variables, a few from the variable `COPD`, while many are missing from `LOS`. Missing observations are coloured in red, while all completed observations are in green. Overall, our dataset `MMstat` is missing 4% of data.

A small percentage of missing values may not substantially affect the analysis. Also, missing values can be replaced. However, the process of replacing missing

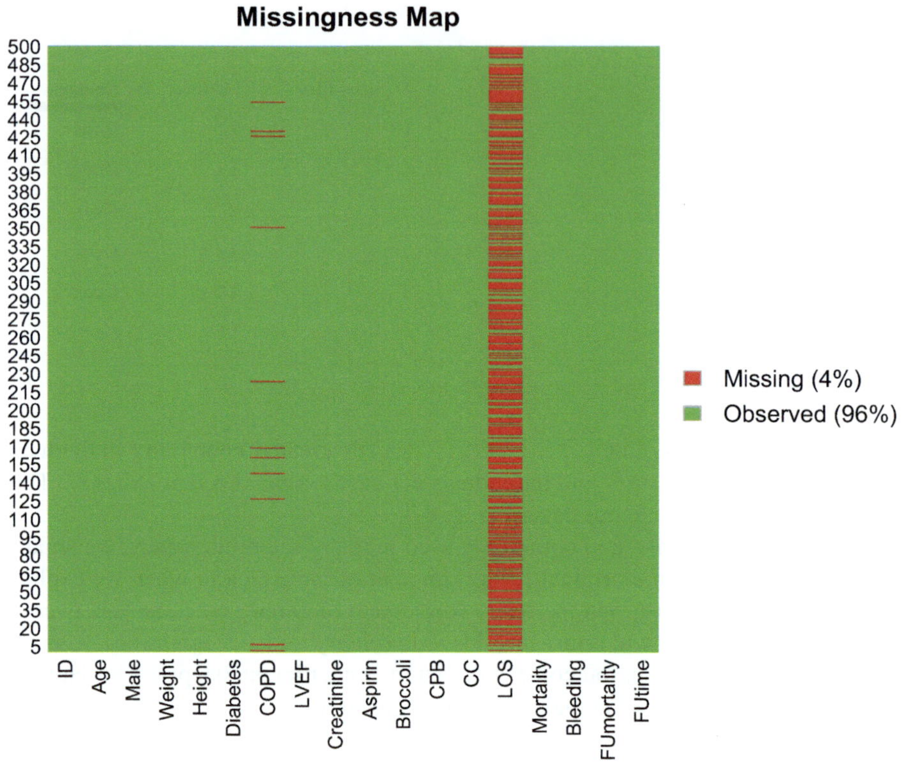

Fig. 4.5 Missingness map from the "Amelia" package

data is complex and is beyond the scope of this book. Later in the book, we discover that if we need to perform propensity score matching analysis (a statistical methodology to create a balanced group), it is not possible in cases where a dataset has missing observations. There are a few techniques to replace missing information. Some are basic, while others are advanced (e.g. multiple imputation). Before proceeding to replace missing variables, we should ask why such observations are missing. Is it intentional or by chance? For continuous values we can fill the gap of missing data by inserting the average. Multiple imputations require advanced statistical knowledge and will not be covered in this book. Nevertheless, the vast majority of "real-world" datasets have missing observations, and it is important to learn how to deal with them.

4.13 The `CreateTableOne` Function

The `CreateTableOne` function from the `tableone` R-package is very handy because it allows us to create relevant tables. Let's use this function to create a table setting out the patients' baseline characteristics. Such a table is often called "table 1" in the majority of scientific papers since it is usually the first table we encounter in manuscripts.

To produce table 1, we must proceed as follows:

1) Convert the variables to factors if we have not done this previously (i.e. we prompt "R" to consider `Male` as a factor, although coded with `0` and `1`, as well as the other factorial variables coded with numbers):

```
> varsToFactor <- c('Male', 'Diabetes', 'Mortality', 'ID',
'Aspirin', 'COPD')
```

2) With the `lapply` function we wrap the new transformed variables to our dataset `MMstat`:

```
> MMstat[varsToFactor] <- lapply(MMstat[varsToFactor], factor)
```

3) We create the object `vars` that contains all the variables (numeric and non-numeric) that we want to include in the table:

```
> vars<- c('Age', 'Weight', 'Height', 'LVEF', 'Creatinine',
'CPB', 'CC', 'Bleeding', 'Male', 'Diabetes', 'Mortality',
'Aspirin', 'LOS', 'COPD')
```

4) Finally, we use the `CreateTableOne` function to create the table. Note that inside the function we must indicate to include the `vars` and `strata` variables, indicating the grouping variable (in this case the `Broccoli` stratum). We also specify that we need the overall (i.e. not grouped) summaries `addOverall = TRUE` as well as the missing values `includeNA = TRUE` (Fig. 4.6).

```
> tableOne <- CreateTableOne(vars = vars, strata = c("Broccoli"),
data = MMstat, addOverall = TRUE, includeNA = TRUE)
> tableOne
```

Note that some variables such as `CPB` and `CC` have a non-normal distribution and should be better presented as median rather than mean as below (Fig. 4.7):

	Stratified by Broccoli Overall	n	y	p	test
n	500	297	203		
Age (mean (SD))	63.23 (12.96)	62.82 (12.81)	63.83 (13.19)	0.392	
Weight (mean (SD))	74.44 (13.89)	74.95 (13.72)	73.68 (14.14)	0.318	
Height (mean (SD))	167.44 (9.24)	168.28 (9.31)	166.20 (9.01)	0.013	
LVEF (mean (SD))	52.65 (8.05)	52.11 (8.65)	53.44 (7.02)	0.071	
Creatinine (mean (SD))	0.88 (0.29)	0.89 (0.29)	0.88 (0.29)	0.629	
CPB (mean (SD))	73.32 (28.61)	80.15 (32.63)	63.31 (17.11)	<0.001	
CC (mean (SD))	40.97 (18.81)	44.78 (20.74)	35.39 (13.84)	<0.001	
Bleeding (mean (SD))	538.53 (172.43)	581.70 (191.09)	475.38 (114.85)	<0.001	
Male = 1 (%)	224 (44.8)	139 (46.8)	85 (41.9)	0.319	
Diabetes (%)				0.550	
0	413 (82.6)	247 (83.2)	166 (81.8)		
1	71 (14.2)	39 (13.1)	32 (15.8)		
2	16 (3.2)	11 (3.7)	5 (2.5)		
Mortality = 1 (%)	44 (8.8)	39 (13.1)	5 (2.5)	<0.001	
Aspirin = 1 (%)	329 (65.8)	217 (73.1)	112 (55.2)	<0.001	
LOS (mean (SD))	14.72 (10.09)	15.34 (8.97)	13.77 (11.60)	0.314	
COPD (%)				0.749	
0	460 (92.0)	271 (91.2)	189 (93.1)		
1	29 (5.8)	19 (6.4)	10 (4.9)		
NA	11 (2.2)	7 (2.4)	4 (2.0)		

Fig. 4.6 Table 4.1 created with the function createTableOne, grouped by Broccoli

	Stratified by Broccoli Overall	n	y	p	test
n	500	297	203		
Age (mean (SD))	63.23 (12.96)	62.82 (12.81)	63.83 (13.19)	0.392	
Weight (mean (SD))	74.44 (13.89)	74.95 (13.72)	73.68 (14.14)	0.318	
Height (mean (SD))	167.44 (9.24)	168.28 (9.31)	166.20 (9.01)	0.013	
LVEF (mean (SD))	52.65 (8.05)	52.11 (8.65)	53.44 (7.02)	0.071	
Creatinine (mean (SD))	0.88 (0.29)	0.89 (0.29)	0.88 (0.29)	0.629	
CPB (median [IQR])	67.00 [55.00, 83.00]	73.00 [58.00, 92.00]	60.00 [53.00, 72.00]	<0.001	nonnorm
CC (median [IQR])	35.00 [29.00, 49.00]	39.00 [30.00, 54.00]	33.00 [27.00, 39.00]	<0.001	nonnorm
Bleeding (mean (SD))	538.53 (172.43)	581.70 (191.09)	475.38 (114.85)	<0.001	
Male = 1 (%)	224 (44.8)	139 (46.8)	85 (41.9)	0.319	
Diabetes (%)				0.550	
0	413 (82.6)	247 (83.2)	166 (81.8)		
1	71 (14.2)	39 (13.1)	32 (15.8)		
2	16 (3.2)	11 (3.7)	5 (2.5)		
Mortality = 1 (%)	44 (8.8)	39 (13.1)	5 (2.5)	<0.001	
Aspirin = 1 (%)	329 (65.8)	217 (73.1)	112 (55.2)	<0.001	
LOS (mean (SD))	14.72 (10.09)	15.34 (8.97)	13.77 (11.60)	0.314	
COPD (%)				0.749	
0	460 (92.0)	271 (91.2)	189 (93.1)		
1	29 (5.8)	19 (6.4)	10 (4.9)		
NA	11 (2.2)	7 (2.4)	4 (2.0)		

Fig. 4.7 Table with not normal variables

```
> Nonnormal<-c('CPB', 'CC')
> print(tableOne, nonnormal=Nonnormal)
```

Comparison p-values are printed along with the table. We cover normal distribution and hypothesis testing later in the book. For now, we have obtained our table that includes the pre-operative characteristics and some operative and post-operative details of the patients grouped by `Broccoli`.

We can see that some differences arise. Individuals who included the broccoli dietary regimen were shorter (166.2±9 cm vs 168.2±9.3 cm, `Broccoli=='y'` vs `Broccoli=='n'` respectively, p=0.013), more patients were on `Aspirin` in the `Broccoli=='n'` group and generally both `CPB` and `CC` were shorter in the `Broccoli=='y'` group with a significant reduction in terms of bleeding (p<0.001) in the latter. Finally, more patients died in the `Broccoli=='n'` group.

This descriptive exercise does not clarify the research question: does `Broccoli=='y'` reduce post-operative complications such as bleeding and mortality? It seems that the individuals who included the broccoli dietary regimen `Broccoli=='y'` bled and died less than the `Broccoli=='n'` patients. Yet more patients in the latter group were on `Aspirin` and were exposed to a prolonged operation time that ultimately may increase post-operative complications.

Later in the book we will apply inferential statistics to better understand predictors for post-operative complications while controlling for the other characteristics.

4.14 Conclusion

Understanding the nature of the variables before analysis is mandatory. In this chapter we explore data types and variable definitions and classifications. We also explore the tools to use within "R" to check for data structure and discover how to transform structure, where necessary. The matter of missing data (which frequently happens in medicine) is discussed, as is the importance of identifying it before analysis. Finally, the `tableone` package is introduced as an easy way to produce even the most complex of tables grouped by variables.

Further Readings

Altman DG. Practical statistics for medical research. London: Chapman and Hall; 1991.
Motulsky H. Intuitive biostatistics: a nonmathematical guide to statistical thinking. New York: Oxford University Press; 2010.

Chapter 5
Data Distribution

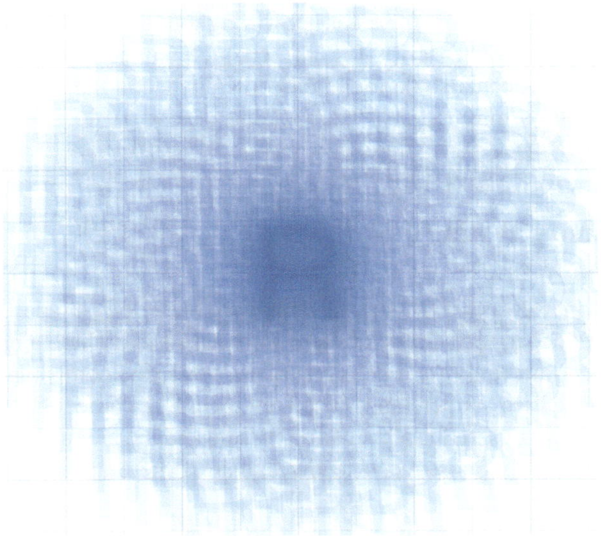

5.1 Software and R-Packages Required for This Chapter

If you haven't already, you need to download and install base-R and R-studio as set out in Chap. 2 under the heading "Downloading "R" and R-studio".

M. Moscarelli, *Biostatistics With 'R': A Guide for Medical Doctors*,
https://doi.org/10.1007/978-3-031-33073-5_5

The relevant R-packages needed for this chapter are:

- epiDisplay—it can be downloaded at:
  http://medipe.psu.ac.th/epicalc
- ggpubr—it can be downloaded at:
  https://rpkgs.datanovia.com/ggpubr/
- tidyverse—it can be downloaded at:
  http://tidyverse.tidyverse.org

5.2 Where to Download the Example Dataset and the Script for This Chapter

If you haven't already downloaded the supplementary dataset named `MMstat.csv` created as a practical example for use throughout this book, you will find it at the link that follows. The script for this chapter named `Chapter 5.Data distribution.R` can also be found and downloaded at the following link:

https://github.com/mmlondon77/Biobook.git

5.3 Normality Testing

Our example dataset `MMstat` has several variables. It is made up of patients undergoing cardiac surgery. Some of them were asked to include a broccoli dietary regimen for a certain timeframe before surgery, while the control group were not. We are interested to understand whether including broccoli, with its anti-inflammatory properties, reduces the mortality rate and the amount of post-operative bleeding of patients. We also want to investigate if there are any other effects at follow-up.

The example dataset has numeric and non-numeric variables which may have some effect on our outcomes of interest (mortality and bleeding) aside from broccoli (e.g. older people may die more frequently after surgery since they are at higher risk, or patients with diabetes and/or who are taking aspirin may bleed more). How do we summarise the patients' baseline characteristics?

The previous Chap. 4 describes how to use the `tableone` R-package to produce and present Table 1 which sets out the patients' baseline characteristics.

However, in order to *summarise* the patients' baseline characteristics, do we use the *mean* or *median*? How do we go about hypothesis testing? Do we use a t-test or something else for the continuous variables?

We will explore the nature of the variables before further analysis, since both summary and inference depend on a variable's distribution. In fact, we need to ascertain if the numerical variables are normally distributed or may follow a different data distribution. Then we have two paths, graphical visualisation and numerical confirmation with specific testing for normality.

Remember normal distribution only makes sense for numerical data (i.e. there is no need to investigate normality distribution for categorical, non-numeric, qualitative data).

This chapter also describes how to use the following graphics for plotting continuous variables and inspecting for normality:

- Histogram
- Q-Q plot and density plot
- Boxplot

Interchangeably, graphics will be coded with basic graphic from base-R (basic graphic) as well as more advanced packages such as `ggplot2`.

5.4 Histogram

Any data sample will form a distribution. Distribution provides mathematical function that can be used to calculate the probability for any individual observation from the sample space.

By far the most well-known distribution is the Gaussian distribution (the standard normal distribution).

First, we can create a normal distribution, to set the foundation and show the "perfect normal plot" (standard normal distribution/bell-shaped Gaussian curve).

```
> x = seq(-15, 15, by=0.1)
> y = dnorm(x, mean(x), sd(x))
> plot(x,y, col='red', ylab='', xlab='', axes=FALSE, main='The
normal distribution', lwd=3, type='l')
```

You can use the code above to obtain the curve shown below that has a certain given mean and standard deviation (Fig. 5.1):

Next, we can produce a histogram with a similar normality shape (Fig. 5.2):

```
x <- rnorm(10000, mean=90, sd=5)
hist(x, breaks=50)
truehist(x, axes=FALSE, ylab='', xlab='')#from the library MASS
lines(density(x))
```

We won't break down the code above just yet; this is only to show you how a normal distribution should look when plotted as a histogram.

Now, let us investigate if numeric covariates of our dataset have the same similar shape. We start with the covariate `Age` (overall cohort, broccoli and control).

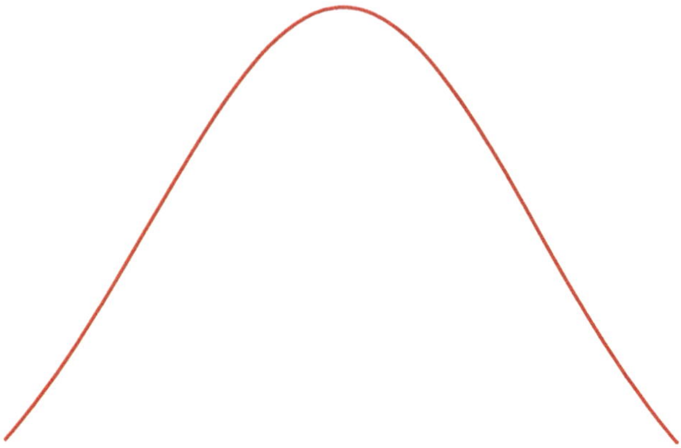

Fig. 5.1 The shape of normal distribution

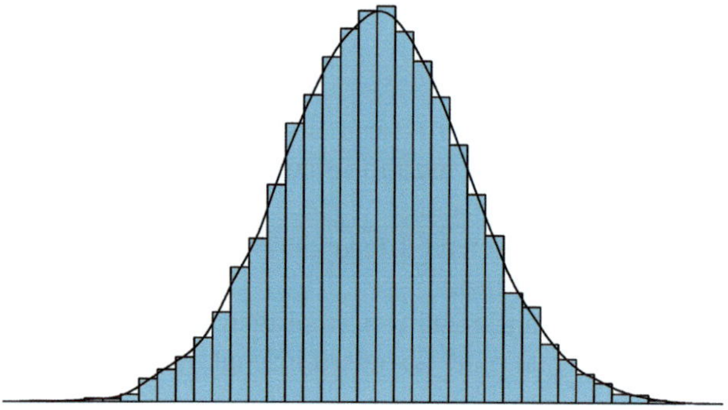

Fig. 5.2 Histogram showing normal distribution

```
> hist(MMstat$Age, main='Age distribution, overall cohort',
col='lightblue', xlab='Age years old')
```

For this the function `hist( )` is used to plot the age distribution of the overall cohort as a histogram (Fig. 5.3).

Does it look similar to the normal histogram shown before? No, it does not. The distribution is definitely not normal and left skewed from the presence of outliers on the left side of the distribution and towards the left tail. Frankly, there is no bell-shaped curve.

Now we plot two other distributions, cardio-pulmonary bypass (`CPB`) and cross-clamp/ischaemic time (`CC`) for further analysis and comparison (Fig. 5.4):

Conversely from the left-skewed age distribution, the two variables `CPB` and `CC` are right skewed due to the presence of outliers on the right side of the plotted distribution and towards the right tail this time.

We see that, for summary purposes in these cases, we need to use the median and the range interquartile (the latter is a measure of dispersion). Then for hypothesis testing, we should use a non-parametric test. However, later on in the book we will cover measures of central tendency and hypothesis testing. This chapter focuses

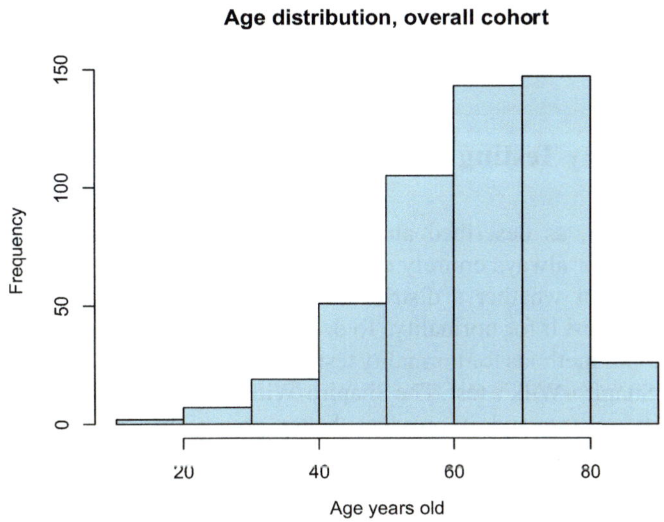

Fig. 5.3 Left-skewed data distribution

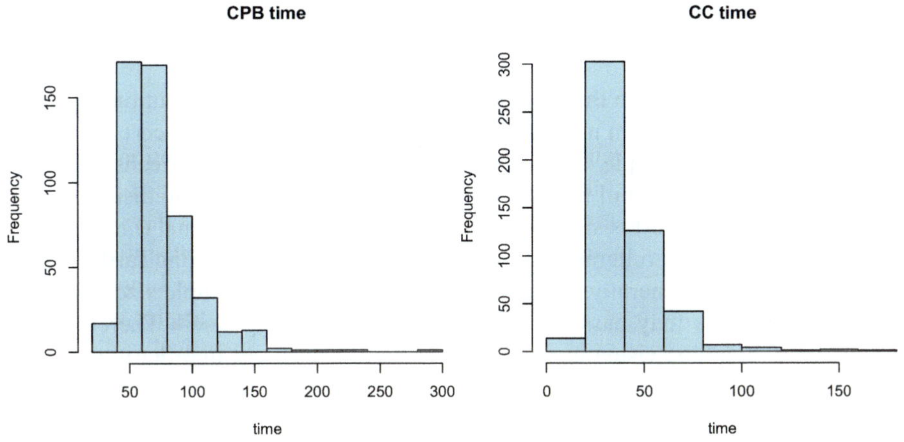

Fig. 5.4 Right-skewed data distribution

only on data distribution and how to discriminate between normal and non-normal distribution.

5.5 Normality Testing

Visual inspection, as described above, remains pivotal yet may sometimes be deceiving. It is not always entirely clear how skewed a plot is. In order to reach a proper decision of whether a distribution is normal (bell-shaped Gaussian), we should formally test it for normality. To do so we must find the p-value.

There are two methods for normality testing: the Kolmogorov-Smirnov normality test and the Shapiro-Wilk's test. The Shapiro-Wilk's method is highly recommended for normality testing and it provides better power than Kolmogorov-Smirnov normality test. It is based on the correlation between the data and the corresponding normal scores. We can run the Shapiro-Wilk's test using the formula below:

```
> shapiro.test(MMstat$Age)
    Shapiro-Wilk normality test
data:   MMstat$Age
W = 0.95696, p-value <0.001
```

Take into consideration that any p-value <0.05 tells us the distribution of data is significantly different from normal distribution. From this we can ascertain that the p-value from our example dataset is highly significant, which means we can't assume normality! The null hypothesis of the test is that the sample distribution is normal. Hence if the test is significant, the distribution is non-normal (i.e. we reject the null hypothesis). I reiterate that we investigate hypothesis testing further in the book. Do note that generally, normality tests are sensitive to sample size. Meaning small sample sizes may pass normality tests, just for being small. Therefore, it's important to combine visual inspection and a significance test in order to make the right decision. It is important to also keep in mind that for the Shapiro-Wilk's test, missing values are allowed, but the number of non-missing values must be between 3 and 5000.

5.6 More About Visual Inspection with Regard to Normality

As already outlined, visual inspection brings to life many details, yet there are no numbers (i.e. there is no hypothesis testing). In the example above we want to understand the `Age` of our study sample (n=500, the overall cohort) follows a normal distribution. Since the Shapiro-Wilk's test rejected the hypothesis of normality, we should assume that the covariate `Age` follows a non-normal (skewed) distribution.

At this point (aside from the histogram) we can use two further methods to inspect normality. The first is:

- *Q-Q plot*: Q-Q stands for "quantile-quantile" and draws the correlation between a given sample and the normal distribution. A 45-degree reference line is also plotted.
- Let us use the `epiDisplay` R-package with the `shapiro.qqnorm( )` function (Fig. 5.5):

```
> library(epiDisplay)
> shapiro.qqnorm(MMstat$Age)
```

All the observations (i.e. the circles) should be sitting on the dotted blue line. However, both tails of the distribution, in particularly, are moving away from the reference line. The Shapiro-Wilk's test output ($p<0.001$) is also reported. Together they suggest violation of normality distribution.

A more aesthetically elegant way to visualise the Q-Q plot would be by using the `ggpubr` R-package (the "gg" stands for grammar of graphic) (Fig. 5.6):

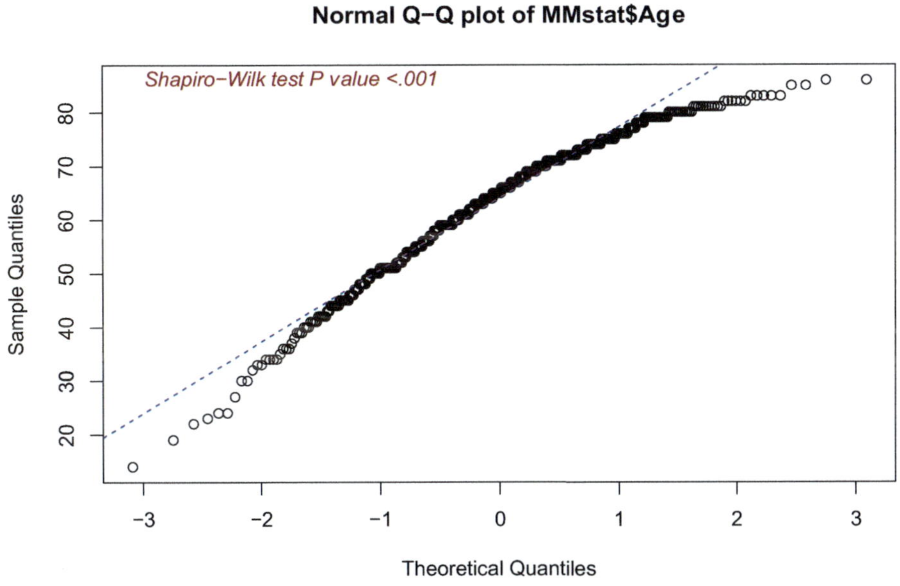

Fig. 5.5 Q-Q (quantile-quantile) plot to assess normality

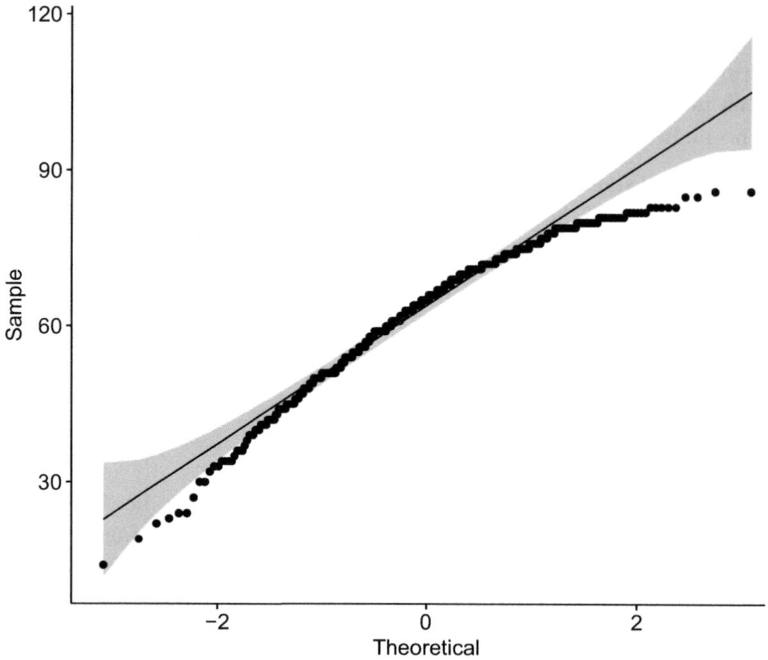

Fig. 5.6 Elegant way for Q-Q plot with 95% confidence interval

```
> library(ggpubr)
> ggqqplot(MMstat$Age)
```

All values are plotted along the 95% confidence interval. Later in the book we will address the confidence interval in more detail. For the time being, values are plotted along with their variability (grey shadow).

The second method to inspect for normality is (Fig. 5.7):

- *Density plot:* for which we use the `ggpubr` R-package again:

```
> ggdensity(MMstat$Age, main = "Density plot of Age whole
cohort", xlab = "Age", col='darkgreen', lwd=2)
```

Looking at the density plot above, it is intuitive that the distribution is "left skewed" due to outliers, in our case some patients with young ages. The density plot basically resembles the shape of the histogram.

Some embellishment was added to the code for the density plot. The embellishment makes a plot more aesthetically pleasing and also more meaningful and informative.

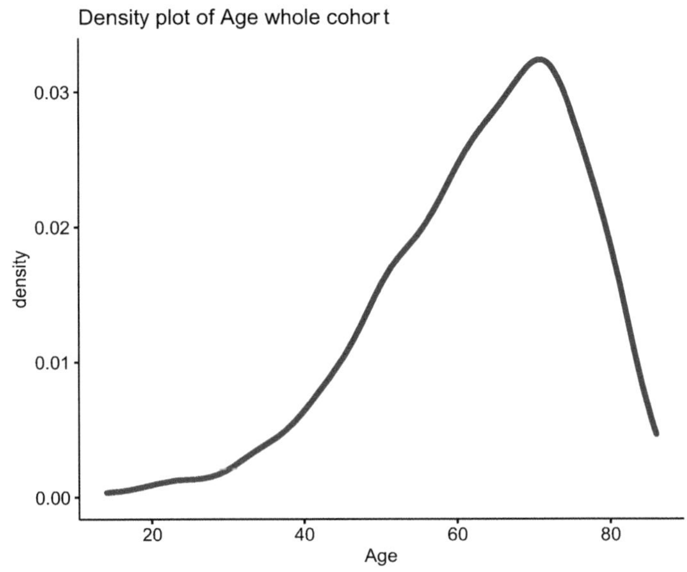

Fig. 5.7 Density plot of age

- `main`—adds a title to the plot
- `xlab`—assigns a name to the x-axis
- `col`—assigns a colour to the density line
- `lwd`—adjusts the plot line width (we used `lwd=2`, you can experiment with different widths to see what happens)

5.7 Do We Need to Test for Normality in All Cases?

Yes, normality tests are always required. However, if the sample size is large enough (i.e. $n > 30$), we may ignore data distribution tests and use a parametric test (tests for normally distributed values) instead. The central limit theorem outlines that no matter what distribution things have, the sampling distribution tends to be normal if our sample is large enough ($n > 30$). Nevertheless, we should always check for normality.

As a rule of thumb, if a distribution has a certain mean and a standard deviation (standard deviation demonstrates the spread or variability of the data) higher than 1/3 of the mean, the distribution is not normal (e.g. the mean is 60 with a standard deviation of 28). Therefore, we should represent the data with the median and interquartile range.

5.8 Central Limit Theory

Having already been introduced to the standard normal distribution, it is now time to understand better the central limit theorem. The normal distribution is in fact important because of the central limit theorem.

The theorem states that the population of all possible sample sizes (n) from a population with a mean (μ) and a variance (σ^2) approaches a normal distribution with μ and σ^2/n when n approaches infinity.

We can therefore assume that the variable `Age` has a normal distribution, considering the sample size is very large ($n = 500$) with no missing data. We know that the mean `Age` with standard deviation of the whole cohort is:

```
> mean(MMstat$Age)
[1] 63.2
> sd(MMstat$Age)
[1] 12.96
```

What is the percentage of individuals with age higher than 80 in the sample?

We apply the function `pnorm( )` for the assumed normal distribution with mean 63.2 and standard deviation 12.9. Since we are looking for the percentage of patients with age scoring higher than 80, we are interested in the upper tail of the normal distribution.

```
> pnorm(80, mean=63.2, sd=12.9, lower.tail=FALSE)
[1] 0.09640256
```

This tells us the percentage of individuals with age greater than 80 in the whole cohort is 9.6%.

5.9 Properties of Normal Distribution

Some facts about normal distribution:

1. The mean, mode and median are all equal (mean, median and mode are central tendency indices).
2. The curve is symmetric at the centre (i.e. at the mean) whereby exactly half of the values are to the left of centre and the other half of the values are to the right.
3. The total area under the curve is equal to 1.
4. 68% of the data has a standard deviation of 1 or less.
5. 95% of the data has a standard deviation of 2 or less.
6. 99.7% of the data has a standard deviation of 3 or less.

5.10 Subsetting for Normality Testing

Does Age distribution differ in the broccoli vs noBroccoli groups? To answer this we must plot the Age distribution grouped by broccoli vs noBroccoli. But before that, we must first split the dataset into broccoli and noBroccoli individuals. To split the dataset, we in fact subset the dataset, creating chunks. Subsetting is the process of retrieving certain parts of the data which are of interest for a specific purpose. Subsetting is explained in greater detail in Chap. 3. Hereinafter follows a partial overview for the purposes of this section.

We use the following code with base-R:

```
> Broccoli<-MMstat[MMstat$Broccoli=='y',]
```

The code will create the Broccoli object that contains only the information about individuals who include the broccoli dietary regimen before surgery. The brackets [ ] in this case are used for subsetting. It is important to note that 'y' is in between single speech marks and refers to the level specification of the broccoli variable that was coded as either y or n. Also "=" in "R" is used to assign an element to a vector, equal to the arrow <-. "==" in "R" is used to represent the meaning of equality in a mathematical sense. In this case the Broccoli object should equal/ include == all the elements with broccoli 'y'.

It is also important to note that the comma before the end of the square brackets ,] specifies that all columns must be imported into the subset.

Now we create the noBroccoli group:

```
> noBroccoli<-MMstat[MMstat$Broccoli=='n',]
```

Here we specify to assign all the information about Broccoli=='n' patients to the noBroccoli subset. Once we have created the two objects containing all information about Broccoli patients and noBroccoli patients, let us hist( ) them both to inspect for distribution:

```
> hist(noBroccoli$Age, main='Age distribution Broccoli vs no
Broccoli', xlab='Age years old', col='lightgreen', ylim=c(0,80))
> x<-hist(Broccoli$Age, add=T)
```

We enter into the code the plot name main=, the x-axis name xlab=, the colour of the histogram some bins col= and the limits of the y-axis ylim=c( ) (Fig. 5.8).

It is intuitive that both age distributions, Broccoli and noBroccoli, have non-normal right-skewed distribution.

We can also achieve subsetting using the dplyr function from the tidyverse R-package as explained in Chap. 3:

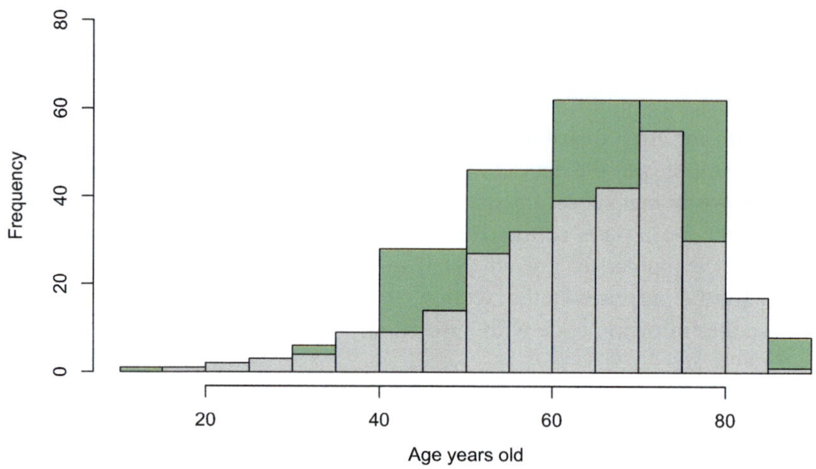

Fig. 5.8 Age distribution of Broccoli vs noBroccoli

```
> Broccoli<-filter(MMstat, Broccoli=='y')
> noBroccoli<-filter(MMstat, Broccoli=='n')
```

5.11 Hint from the Grammar of Graphic

Plotting in "R" can be performed with basic graphic (as the histogram in Fig. 5.8) or with higher-level graphic such as grammar of graphic. Grammar of graphic is a grammar used "to describe and create a wide range of statistical graphics". The layered grammar of graphics approach is implemented in the `ggplot2` R-package. Layered means that the plot is created adding layer over layer. This is further clarified later in this chapter.

Another higher-level package for graphics is `lattice`; however, it is not covered in full in this book, but just few examples.

In this chapter, and generally throughout this book, plots are produced interchangeably with basic graphic and `ggplot2`.

Let us delve more into `ggplot2`.

This paragraph can be skipped without losing information; however, it is good to view the code which produces the following plot because it automatically divides the age results for `Broccoli` and `noBroccoli` patients and also shows the mean of each group represented as dotted lines (Fig. 5.9).

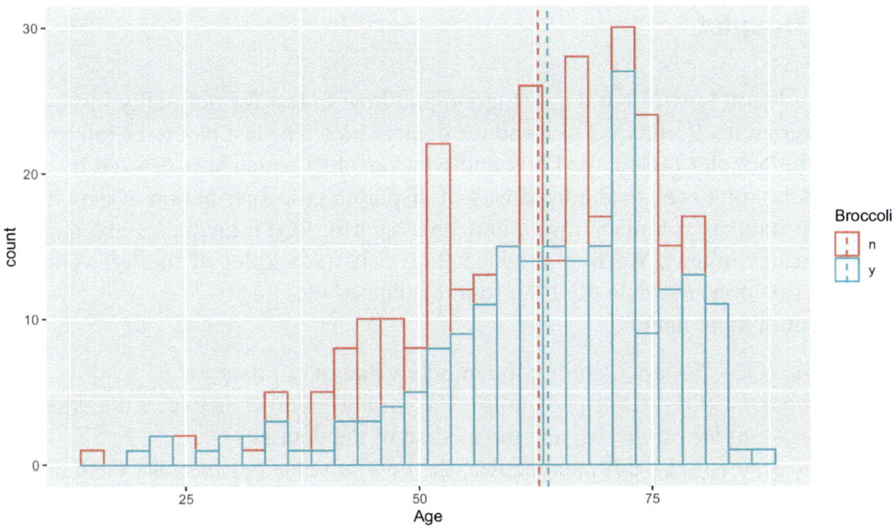

Fig. 5.9 Age grouped by the Broccoli variable, with mean age depicted as red and green dotted lines

```
> library(plyr) # Opening the library plyr
> mu <- ddply(MMstat, "Broccoli", summarise, grp.mean=mean(Age))
#Creating the mean of the Broccoli and no-Broccoli subgroups
> head(mu) #Visualizing the mean

  Broccoli grp.mean
1        n 62.82155
2        y 63.83251

> x<-ggplot(MMstat, aes(x=Age, color=Broccoli, fill=Broccoli)) +
   geom_histogram(position="identity", alpha=0.5) #Creating the
object 'x' as histogram according to Broccoli / no-Broccoli

> x+geom_vline(data=mu, aes(xintercept=grp.mean, color=Broccoli),
             linetype="dashed") # adding the mean (dotted lines)
```

The coding for ggplot2 looks very intimidating and difficult to digest and master for beginners. However, this advanced form of plotting helps us to automatically subset the dataset and visualise the chunks. It is also very important and helpful for the data exploratory analysis process.

Explaining how ggplot2 works *in detail* is beyond the scope of this book. However, a superficial overview is provided which should get you practicing it enough to eventually discover how powerful it is. Graphs bring data to life!

The next section sets out more detailed examples on how to produce plots in both basic graphic and ggplot2.

5.12 Boxplot

You have learnt how to build a histogram and how to test for normality inspecting the histogram itself, the Q-Q plot and the density plot. The last plot to be introduced here is the boxplot (also called box and whisker plot) which was devised by John Tukey. A boxplot is a standardised way of displaying the distribution of data based on a five-number summary (minimum, first quartile (Q1), median, third quartile (Q3) and maximum). We now produce (Fig. 5.10) a boxplot of the left ventricle ejection function covariate (`LVEF`) from the dataset `MMstat`:

Set out in more detail:

- *median* (Q2—50th percentile): the middle value of our dataset
- *first quartile* (Q1—25th percentile): the middle number between the smallest number (*not the minimum*) and the median of the dataset
- *third quartile* (Q3—75th percentile): the middle value between the median and the highest value (*not the maximum*) of the dataset
- *interquartile range* (IQR): 25th to the 75th percentile
- *whiskers* (vertical dotted black line)
- *outliers*
- *maximum*: Q3 + 1.5*IQR
- *minimum*: Q1 -1.5*IQR

Boxplot is a very nice way to represent numbers. It shows you at glance "strange" numbers (outliers). An asymmetric boxplot may indicate a non-normal distribution. From the plot of `LVEF`, we can note a few outliers. The definition of outliers is somewhat arbitrary. Just as arbitrary is the definition of minimum and maximum in the boxplot. The minimum is calculated as Q1 - 1.5*IQR and the maximum as

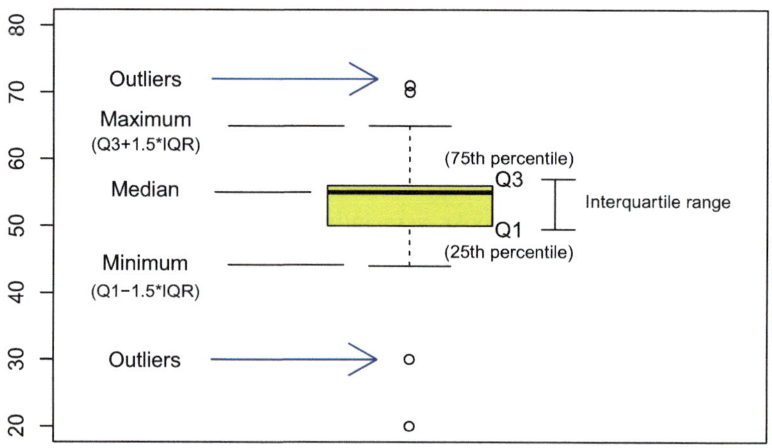

Fig. 5.10 Boxplot for left ventricle ejection function (LVEF)

Q3 - 1.5*IQR; hence, they are not the smallest or highest numbers in the boxplot. Rather they establish a cutoff above and below for which we can define numbers as outliers. In essence, an outlier is a conventional definition of the minimum and the maximum. It is pivotal to spot outliers since it may provide very important information. They can be data entry errors or uncommon values. Sometimes we need to remove them when we carry out calculations (e.g. in regression they may affect and influence the result very aggressively). Other times they do not significantly affect the output and we can keep them. Nevertheless, it is very important to understand them.

Is the `LVEF` normally distributed? Let us plot all the `LVEF` graphics at once (Fig. 5.11):

```
> par(mfrow=c(2,2))
> hist(MMstat$LVEF, col='yellow', xlab='LVEF%', main='LVEF histogram')
> boxplot(MMstat$LVEF, col='green', main= 'LVEF boxplot', boxwex=0.5)
> shapiro.qqnorm(MMstat$LVEF, title='Q-Q')
```

As well as the density plot (Fig. 5.12):

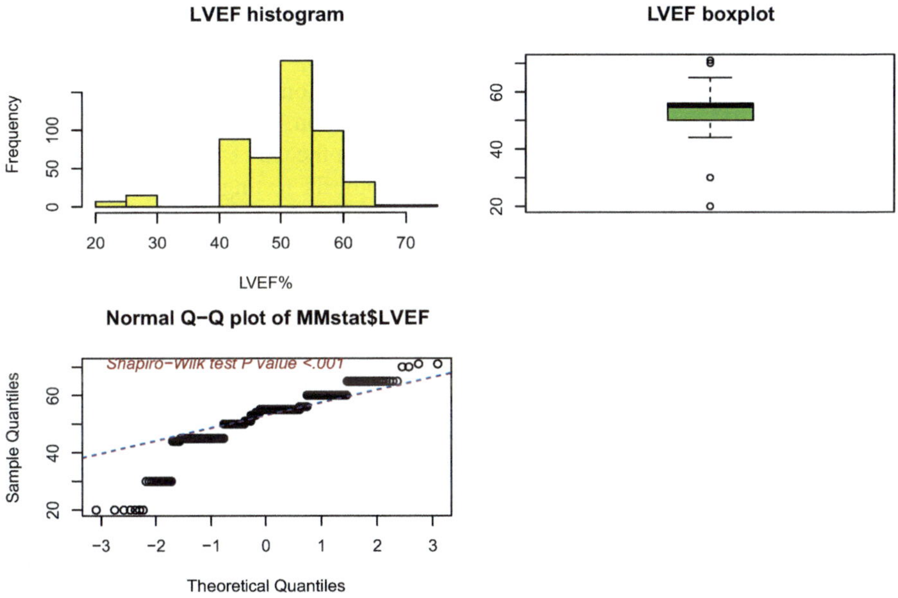

Fig. 5.11 Histogram, boxplot and Q-Q plot for left ventricle ejection function (LVEF)

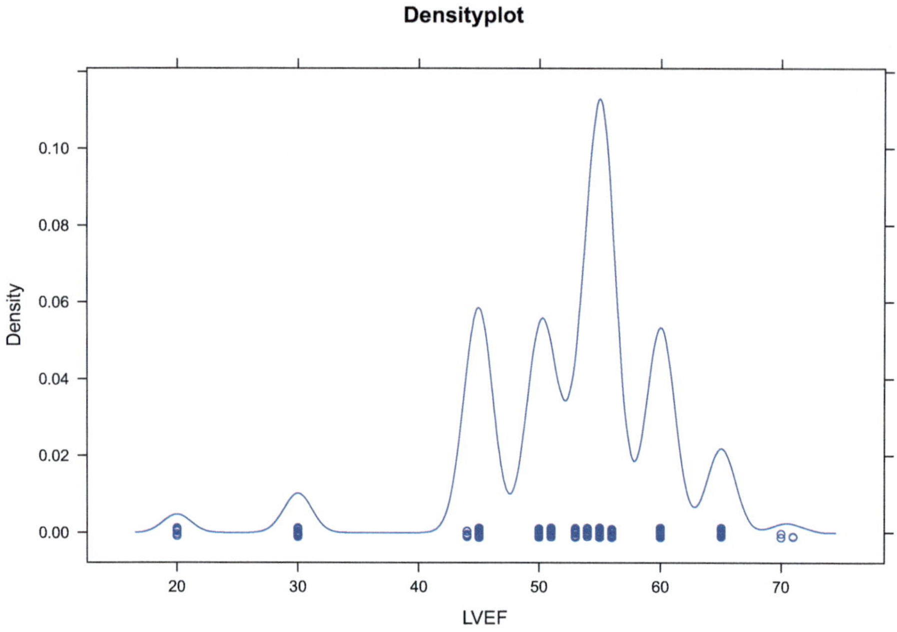

Fig. 5.12 Density plot for left ventricle ejection function (LVEF)

```
> densityplot(MMstat$LVEF, xlab='LVEF', main='Densityplot')
```

Clearly, the `LVEF` does not have a normal distribution (Shapiro test <0.001) and should be summarised as median and standard deviation. Notably, for the last visual tool, we use the `densityplot( )` function from the `lattice` R-package.

Boxplot is very useful for visualising hypothesis testing from two or more groups. Let us plot the age distribution of the Broccoli vs noBroccoli groups using basic graphic (Fig. 5.13):

```
> boxplot(MMstat$Age~MMstat$Broccoli, col=c('lightgreen', 'dark-
green'), main='Age Broccoli vs no-Broccoli', ylim=c(0,100), box-
wex=0.5, xlab='Group: Broccoli=y, no-Broccoli=n', ylab='Age y/o')
```

It is easy to see that the median and the spread around it are not very different between the two groups, except with more outliers in the `noBroccoli` group.

Let us see what happens if we plot the same data using `ggplot2` instead of basic graphic (Fig. 5.14):

This plot is very informative. Not only does it show the five numbers of the boxplot, but also every single observation is plotted. Now we can see clearer how many patients are in each group. In fact, the "jittering" is one way to display the sample size. Notably this information is not incorporated in the boxplot created using basic graphic.

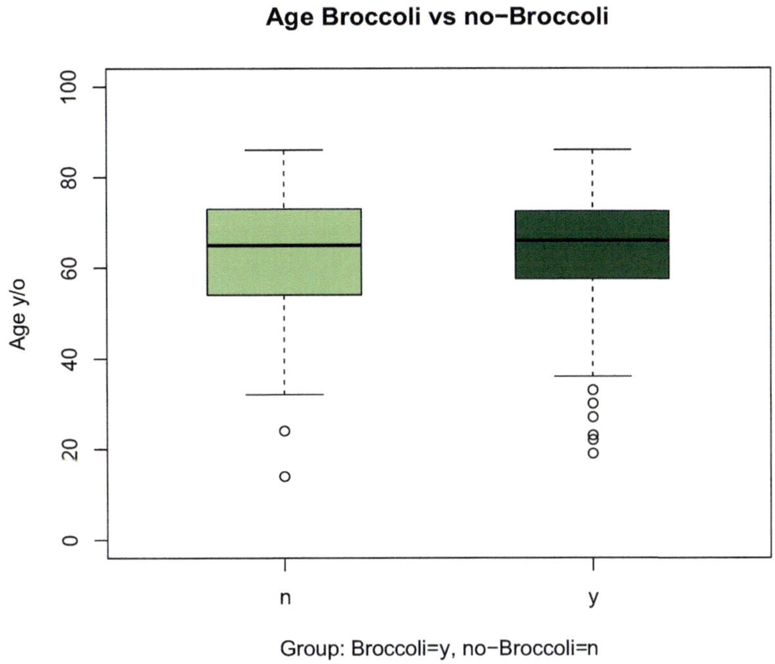

Fig. 5.13 Boxplot of age grouped by Broccoli vs noBroccoli using basic graphic

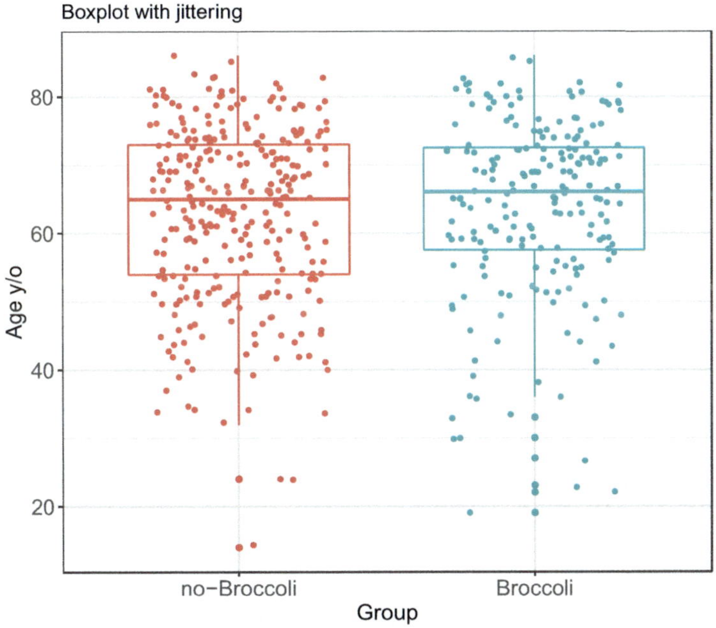

Fig. 5.14 Boxplot of age grouped by Broccoli vs noBroccoli using ggplot2

The code used is discussed in small detail below; however, it may take time to master ggplot2 and it probably needs an entire book explaining how to use it properly:

```
# Create Elegant Data Visualisations Using the Grammar of Graphics
> ggplot(MMstat, aes(x=Broccoli, y=Age, color=Broccoli)) +theme_
bw()+ geom_boxplot() + geom_jitter(shape = 16, position=position_
jitter(0.3)) +xlab("Group") + ylab("Age y/o")+labs(title='Boxplot
with jittering')+theme(axis.title.x = element_text(size=14),axis.
text.x = element_text(size=14), axis.text.y=element_
text(size=14),axis.title.y=element_text(size=14), legend.position
= "none")+ scale_x_discrete(labels=c("n" = "no-Broccoli", "y" =
"Broccoli"))
```

The code works as you are adding layers to it:

ggplot(MMstat [we use the general function ggplot and apply it to our dataset MMstat] aes(x=Broccoli, y=Age, color=Broccoli)) [sets out to plot Broccoli vs noBroccoli on the x-axis and Age on the y-axis, also to fill the plot with Age data for each Broccoli and noBroccoli individual] +theme_bw()+ geom_boxplot() + geom_jitter(shape = 16, position=position_jitter(0.3)) [specifies to display the plot with a standard theme of black and to present the data about Broccoli vs noBroccoli with both boxplot and jitter and also specifies the shape and size of the dots (in this case jitter provides a nice visualisation of the population of each Broccoli and noBroccoli subset)] +xlab("Group") + ylab("Age y/o")+labs(title='Boxplot with jittering')+theme(axis.title.x = element_text(size=14),axis.text.x = element text(size=14), axis.text.y=element_text(size=14),
axis.title.y=element_text(size=14) [outlines the names of the x-axis ("Group"), y-axis ("Age y/o"), the main title of the graphic ("Boxplot with jittering") and the size of the characters (size=...)] legend.position = "none")[removes the legend, for aesthetic reasons] + scale_x_discrete(labels=c("n" = "no-Broccoli", "y" = "Broccoli")) [partitions the x-lab into Broccoli and noBroccoli].

You should practice with the example dataset. It takes some time, but at the end of the day it will be rewarding. Always remember that "R" language is case sensitive; any small typo will affect the code. The table below may help you understand how the plot is produced adding layer by layer:

first layer	
ggplot( )	Every ggplot2 graph starts with the function ggplot

`ggplot(MMstat, )`	The dataset containing all variables must be specified at first
`ggplot(MMstat, aes(x=Broccoli, y=Age, color=Broccoli))`	Aesthetics can be added (e.g. for the x-axis `x=Broccoli`, for the y-axis `y=Age`) and colour specification (e.g. `color=Broccoli`) is also added here
+ *second layer*	
`+theme_bw()`	Next add a theme; in this case a black and white theme (`theme_bw()`) was used, but there are many others
+ *third layer and fourth*	
`+geom_boxplot() + geom_jitter(shape = 16, position=position_jitter(0.3))`	Then comes the *geom* functions which add the layers of plotting on the coordinate system, according to its geometry; in our case we selected boxplot `geom_boxplot()` and jittering `geom_jitter( )`, specifying shapes and position of the jitters
+ *sixth and seventh layer*	
`+xlab("Group") + ylab("Age y/o")`	Labels for the x- and y-axes are specified
+ *eighth*	
`+labs(title='Boxplot with jittering')`	Title for the plot is entered
+ *ninth layer*	
`+theme(axis.title.x = element_text(size=14),axis.text.x = element_text(size=14), axis.text.y=element_text(size=14), axis.title.y=element_text(size=14), legend.position = "none")`	This specifies the axis theme, where the title and text size (size=14) of the labels of both x- and y-axes are specified, and the legend is removed
+ *tenth layer*	
`+ scale_x_discrete(labels=c("n" = "no-Broccoli", "y" = "Broccoli"))`	Adds names to the groups along the x-axis

5.13 How to Treat Non-numeric Variables

As examples, take `Diabetes` which has three levels (0=no diabetes, 1=non-insulin dependent, 2=insulin dependent) or `Male` which has two levels (0=female, 1=male); we should not check for normality or hypothesis test them. Instead we should use the chi-squared test. Chi-squared is a non-parametric statistic, also called a distribution-free test. Non-parametric tests should be used when the level of measurement of the variable is nominal or ordinal (i.e. non-numeric).

5.14 Plotting Categorical Variables

This section shows how to plot non-numeric categorical (ordinal) variables. Say we would like to depict the proportion of patients in the diabetic class. As outlined above, the `Diabetes` covariate has three levels: 0, 1 and 2 which stand for no diabetes, non-insulin-dependent diabetes mellitus (NIDDM) and insulin-dependent diabetes mellitus, respectively. We have already transformed the variable from class numerical to factorial in Chap. 4 of this book. The class `Diabetes` is ordinal, since the three levels have different biological effects on patients (IDDM is obviously more detrimental than the NIDDM and not having diabetes at all). We cannot use the `boxplot` function, nor the `hist` function. It is better to use the function (Fig. 5.15) `barplot`:

```
> class<-c('no-Broccoli', 'Broccoli')
>   barplot(table(MMstat$Diabetes,MMstat$Broccoli),main='Diabetic
patients', col=c('lightgreen', 'yellow', 'red'), ylim=c(0,400),
ylab='Number',names.arg=class, beside=TRUE, border=NA)
> legend("topright", c('none', 'NIDDM', 'IDDM'), bty='n',lty=c(1,1),
lwd=3, col=c('lightgreen', 'yellow', 'red'),cex=1.5)
```

This is created using basic graphic functionality. As mentioned earlier, this book jumps between basic graphic and `ggplot2`. The function `barplot` is used in order to show the distribution of the proportion of diabetic patients in both `Broccoli` vs `noBroccoli` groups. To do so we use the `barplot` function, followed by the `table(MMstat$Diabetes,MMstat$Broccoli)` function. The `table` function returns the number of patients in each group.

```
> table(MMstat$Diabetes, MMstat$Broccoli)


      n   y
  0 247 166
  1  39  32
  2  11   5
```

`Broccoli` patients are specified by the column `y` (=166+32+5) and `noBroccoli` patients by the column `n` (247+39+11). The rows set out the numbers of non-diabetic (level=0), NIDDM (level=1) and IDDM (level=2) in each group (y/n). Basically, we use the function `barplot` to plot this table. All other arguments are embellishment.

Notably, as you can see from Fig. 5.15, `barplot` can be portrayed as stacked bars (depicted on the right, argument `beside` =FALSE) or as juxtaposed bars (depicted on the left, argument `beside` =TRUE).

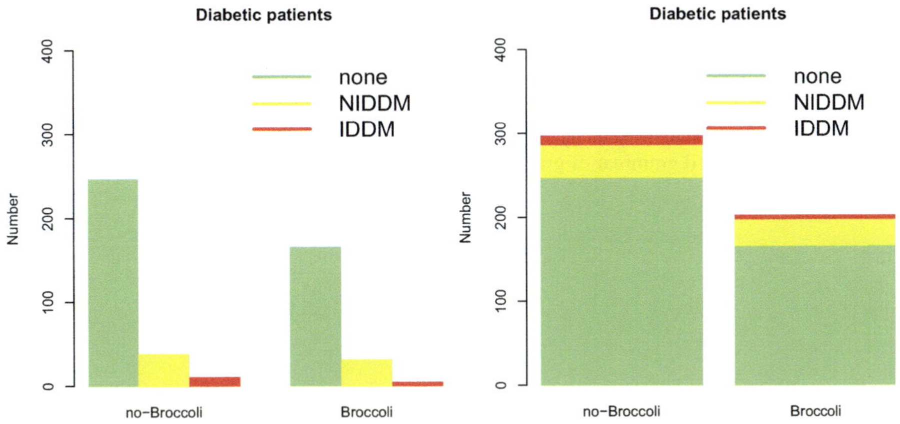

Fig. 5.15 Barplot distribution of diabetes (three levels) grouped by Broccoli vs noBroccoli

5.15 Conclusion

At the incipit of statistical paragraphs of a majority of scientific papers the words "data is checked for normality before further analysis" are often found. This chapter addresses this process. It defines normality and presents some methodology for assessing the normality distribution of your numeric data. It is important for you to inspect visually the distribution of your numeric data with the function `hist` or `boxplot` followed by the numeric covariate of interest (e.g. age, height, etc. from the example dataset). Those functions will help you to visualise the outliers, but not discard them a priori. Some outliers can be entry errors, some others may represent important information. Revise them from a scientific point of view before any action.

The function `shapiro.test` will return a p-value. If the p-value is above 0.05, you should assume your data is normally distributed. You will learn that a normal distribution can be summarised with a mean and standard deviation, or if a skewed non-normal distribution, with median and range interquartile.

Many statistical tests are based on the assumption of normality; hence, checking for normality is pivotal in order to also understand what statistical test to use (i.e. t-test, Wilcoxon test, etc.).

We discuss that a normal distribution has specific properties and 95% of the data falls within two standard deviations of the mean (the centre). We also know from the central limit theory that large samples tend to have a normal distribution. In essence, scientific studies based on large sample sizes may represent the real world in a more accurate way, since they convey more precise, accurate and less variable information.

This chapter introduces `ggplot2` as one of the most powerful and useful packages for producing elegant plots.

Non-numeric variables do not need normality assessment (e.g. diabetes, broccoli, aspirin, etc. from the example dataset). Instead you can use the function `barplot` to depict proportion within groups of interest.

Further Readings

Quinn G, Keough M. Experimental design and data analysis for biologists. Cambridge: Cambridge University Press; 2002. https://doi.org/10.1017/CBO9780511806384.
Sprinthall RC. Basic statistical analysis. 9th ed. Pearson; 2011, ISBN-13: 978-0205052172.
Wickham H. A layered grammar of graphics. J Comput Graph Stat. 2010;19(1):3–28.

Chapter 6
Precision, Accuracy and Indices of Central Tendency

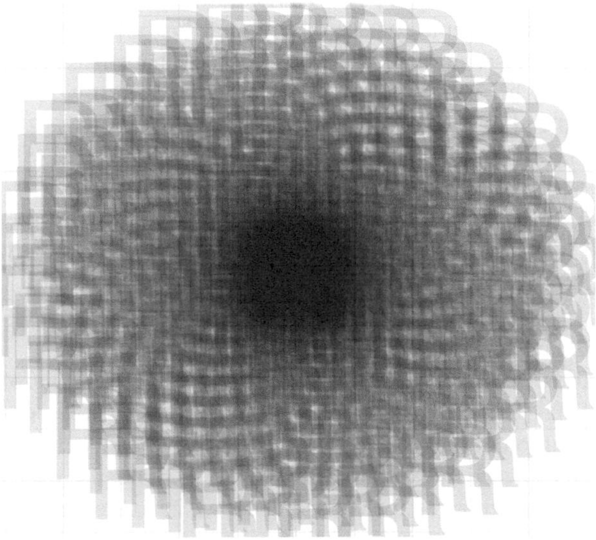

Variance and standard deviation (do not confuse the latter with the standard error of the mean) are measures of variability of a sample. They tell us how far, on average, sample observations lie from the sample mean. The measure of central tendency such as mean, median and mode will also be discussed.

M. Moscarelli, *Biostatistics With 'R': A Guide for Medical Doctors*,
https://doi.org/10.1007/978-3-031-33073-5_6

6.1 Software and R-Packages Required for This Chapter

If you haven't already, you need to download and install base-R and R-studio as set out in Chap. 2 under the heading "Downloading "R" and R-studio".

The relevant R-package needed for this chapter is:

- tidyverse – it can be downloaded at:
  http://tidyverse.tidyverse.org

6.2 Where to Download the Example Dataset and the Script for This Chapter

If you haven't already downloaded the supplementary dataset named MMstat.csv created as a practical example for use throughout this book, you will find it at the link that follows. The script for this chapter named Chapter 6. Precision.R plus an extra supplementary file named Sampledistribution.csv, for use later in this chapter, can also be found and downloaded at the following link:

https://github.com/mmlondon77/Biobook.git

6.3 Precision

What is precision in statistics? Why is precision important?

Precision can be defined as how close a random sample's point of estimate (i.e. the sample mean) is to the one of the true (unknown) population (population mean).

Take the population of the world. It is always unknown since we cannot measure certain variables of every individual in the world (e.g. height, age, etc.). It would take too long, be difficult and expensive. Hence, we can take random samples.

When we take a random sample (n) from a general population (N), the mean of n (defined also as $\bar{x}$) is the best guess of the (unknown) true mean of N (defined also as μ).

Always, n is only an approximate of N; it will never be identical.

When we take random samples from a population, there is always a margin of inevitable error. This error is named standard error of the mean (or simply standard error) and abbreviated as SEM or SE.

However, as a sample size increases, the precision increases. This is something similar (theoretically) to the central limit theory. It is all about sample size!

As a practical example, the variable Age from our example dataset MMstat (which can represent n) is the best guess of the true population age N. N is unknown since it is not measurable.

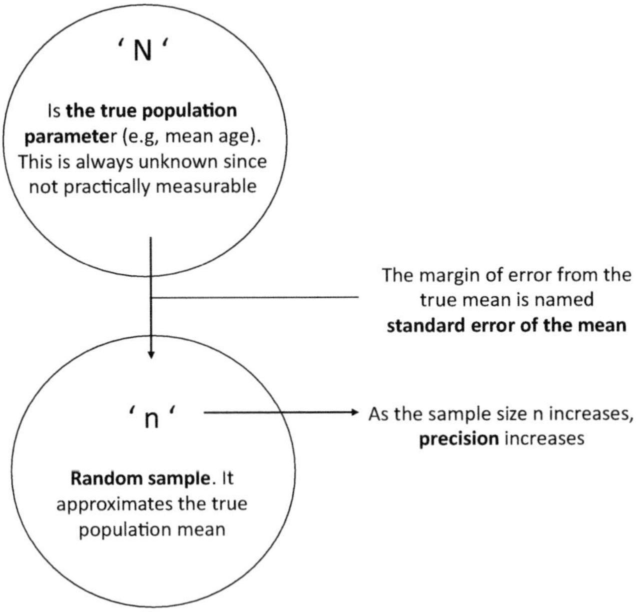

Fig. 6.1 Sample size and precision

The sample n obtained from the general population *N* might be described by a mean value and a measure of dispersion, named standard deviation (SD). But for the moment let's focus on the concept of SE.

Again, SE is a measure of precision and decreases as the sample size increases.

Solid research needs a large sample size. The larger the population included in a study, the more solid the scientific conclusions. A small study can lead to inconclusive and inconsistent results (Fig. 6.1).

6.4 The Relation Between Sample Size and Precision

In order to demonstrate the relation between sample size and precision, we return to normal distribution.

Let's say we want to obtain a true histogram with the code below that uses the function rnorm. The parameters of our fictitious normal population (*N*) are set with a mean of 90 and a SD of 5 (to define normal distribution we need the mean and standard deviation).

```
> x <- rnorm(10000, mean=90, sd=5)
```

We now take many random samples. To do so, we use the function sample to generate random samples from the normal distribution x with replacement replace=TRUE (i.e. anytime a unit is selected, it is replaced in the basket). Importantly all random samples have a size of 10 size=10 and hence are very small.

```
> sample(x, size=10, replace=TRUE)
```

We then calculate the mean of, let's say, 40 random samples ($n = 40$) and build the object sample10.

```
> sample10<-c(90.6, 89, 89, 89.7, 91.5, 89.4, 86.9, 89.2, 89.7,
91.8, 88.7, 88.2, 87.11, 91.2, 91.2, 87.6, 88.9, 91.3, 88.7, 90.4,
89, 90.6, 90, 91.9, 89.3, 91.3, 89.6, 89, 88.1, 89.5, 91.8, 89.7,
88.4, 87.8, 90.1, 89.6, 89.6, 90.7, 89.6, 90.7)
```

Basically, the sample10 object includes each of the means of the 40 random samples. This sample has a grand mean of 89.6 with a standard deviation of 1.3.

We can also do another trial of sampling from the same normal distribution x, this time with a bigger population ($n = 1000$), and perhaps only 24 samples. I will create the object sample1000 that contains the 24 means from a much bigger sample size than sample10.

```
> sample1000(x, size=10000, replace=TRUE)
> sample1000<-c(89.9, 90, 90.2, 90.1, 89.7, 89.8, 90, 89.9, 89.7,
89.8, 90.1, 89.8,90, 90, 89.9, 90, 90, 90, 89.8, 89.9, 89.8,
89.9,89.6)
```

sample1000 has a grand mean of 89.9 with a SD of 0.1.

The SD of these multiple sample means is nothing less than SE. This concept is clarified later in this chapter, where the difference between SE and SD is more clearly outlined.

The purpose now is to graphically represent the distribution of the means of the sample10 and sample1000 objects, with the intent to demonstrate that the variability of a larger sample is less than a smaller sample, and therefore, the precision of a larger sample is higher than that of a smaller sample.

Remember, the larger the sample size, the closer you will get to the true population.

Note that sample1000 has a SD less than sample10.

Let's now plot the two mean distributions, one from the small sample10 and one from the larger sample1000 (Fig. 6.2):

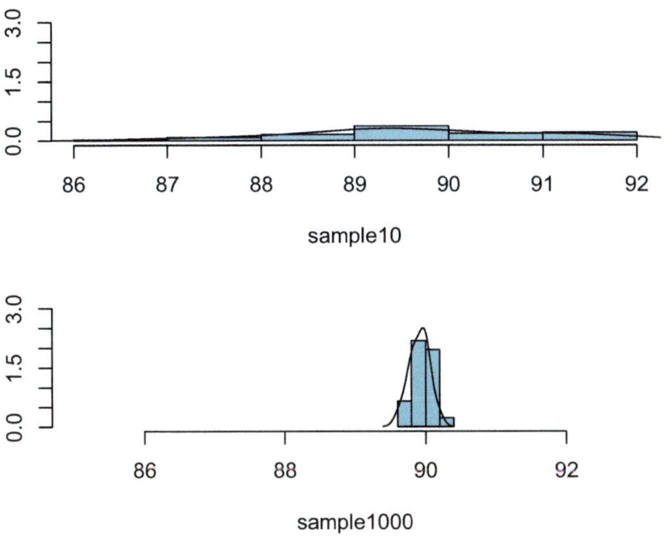

Fig. 6.2 Sampling distribution showing the larger sample size with less variability and spread around the mean

```
> truehist(sample10, ylim=c(0, 3))
> lines(density(sample10))
> truehist(sample1000, ylim=c(0,3), xlim=c(85, 93))
> lines(density(sample1000))
```

Both histograms share the same metrics at the x- and y-axes, but visibly the variability of the larger sample1000 is significantly lower.

Notably both distributions have a similar mean. This clearly demonstrates the importance of plotting distributions. Graphics bring important information to life! Do not just look at numbers.

Let's now plot the two histograms together. This time using ggplot2, as outlined in Chap. 5.

A new .csv file has been created where all values of both objects, sample10 and sample1000, are arranged in a long format. The file is named Sampledistribution.csv and is available for download from GitHub, via the link provided earlier in this chapter.

Long format means data is distributed in one column (opposite to the more usual wide format of different data spread amongst many columns). Many codes in ggplot2 need the data to be in long format as displayed below (Fig. 6.3):

In order to visualise the two mean distributions at once, we use the code below (Fig. 6.4):

Fig. 6.3 Example of data arranged in long format

	A	B	C
1	Sample	mean	
2	Sample10	90.6	
3	Sample10	89	
4	Sample10	89	
5	Sample10	89.7	
6	Sample10	91.5	
7	Sample10	89.4	
8	Sample10	86.9	
9	Sample10	89.2	
10	Sample10	89.7	
11	Sample10	91.8	
12	Sample10	88.7	
13	Sample10	88.2	
14	Sample10	87.11	
15	Sample10	91.2	
16	Sample10	91.2	
17	Sample10	87.6	
18	Sample10	88.9	
19	Sample10	91.3	
20	Sample10	88.7	
21	Sample10	90.4	
22	Sample10	89	
23	Sample10	90.6	
24	Sample10	90	
25	Sample10	91.9	
26	Sample10	89.3	
27	Sample10	91.3	
28	Sample10	89.6	
29	Sample10	89	
30	Sample10	88.1	
31	Sample10	89.5	
32	Sample10	91.8	
33	Sample10	89.7	
34	Sample10	88.4	
35	Sample10	87.8	
36	Sample10	90.1	
37	Sample10	89.6	
38	Sample10	89.6	
39	Sample10	90.7	
40	Sample10	89.6	
41	Sample10	90.7	
42	Sample1000	89.9	
43	Sample1000	90	
44	Sample1000	90.2	
45	Sample1000	90.1	
46	Sample1000	89.7	
47	Sample1000	89.8	
48	Sample1000	90	
49	Sample1000	89.9	
50	Sample1000	89.7	

```
> ggplot(Sampledistribution, aes(mean, fill =Sample)) + geom_
density(alpha = 0.2)
```

As set out in Chap. 5, ggplot2 works in layers:

`ggplot(Sampledistribution [applies the Sampledistribution object to ggplot] aes(mean, fill =Sample)) [adds aesthetics, with the intent to plot the means on the x axis, and each mean represents one of the two samples] + geom_density(alpha = 0.2) [then adds the density function to show the data as a curve with some shading (this style of curve is called alpha)].`

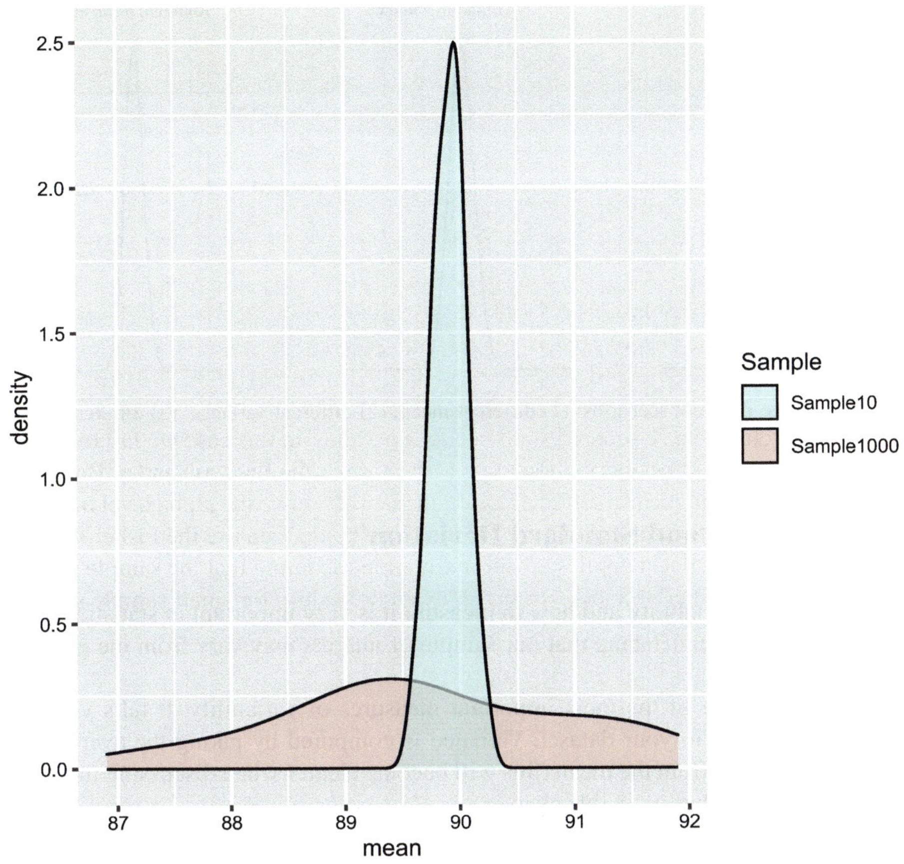

Fig. 6.4 Sampling distribution with ggplot2

Again, this density distribution plot depicts the two distributions along with their very diverse variabilities.

Why is this relevant for medical doctors? Because it demonstrates that more data equals less variability, which is closer to scientific truth.

Now we have explored precision, we can move forward to accuracy. But first, it is important to understand some other concepts of variability (Fig. 6.5).

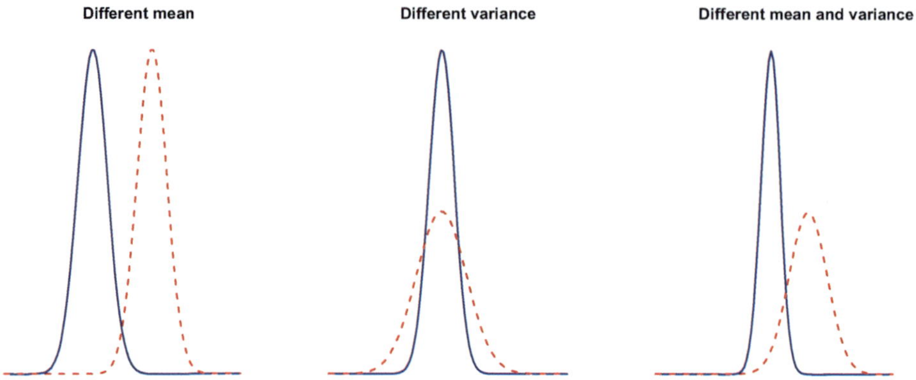

Fig. 6.5 Three different scenarios: (1) different mean, (2) different variance, (3) different mean and variance

6.5 Variance and Standard Deviation

Understanding variability and how to measure it is very important in statistics. It is also important to understand that our sample of interest may vary from the general true population.

Variance is one of the most important measures of variability. It tells you the amount of spread in your dataset. Variance is computed by taking the average of squared deviation from the mean (this will become clearer when discussing the variance equation further on in this chapter).

It is safe to say that the more spread the data has, the larger the variance. It is important to understand that the variance is in relation to the mean (again, it tells you how spread out the data is from the mean).

The SD is derived from the variance. The SD tells you how far each value lies from the mean. It is easy to calculate because it is simply the square root of the variance.

Both the variance and the SD are similar. They reflect the variability in your dataset (the distribution of interest). However, their units differ substantially.

From visualising the sample distribution of sample10 and sample1000, it is clear that the spread is much more evident in the distribution that is smaller in size (i.e. sample10).

The SD is expressed in the same units as the original values (e.g. when analysing the length of the post-operative stay in hospital). The SD will use the unit "number of days" (e.g. 12 ± 2.1 = mean ± SD, which sets out the number of days in hospital as a measure of the length of the post-operative stay).

The variance is expressed in a much larger unit, because the variance is squared.

Considering the unit of a variance is much larger than that used to input information into a dataset, it is harder to interpret the variance intuitively.

Conversely, the SD uses the same units of measure of the population; hence, the SD is easier to understand as a measure of variability.

Nevertheless, the variance is more informative about variability than the SD. Thereby often we need to use the variance in performing statistical inference.

When I say statistical inference, I mean by using the data we have from our sample population, we make a conclusion on the general population as a whole.

6.6 Population and Sample Variance

We can compute two types of "variance" (at least theoretically), the population variance (σ^2) and the sample variance (s^2).

The population variance can be calculated when you have collected all the data from every member of the population that you are interested in. In this very theoretic scenario, you can calculate the exact value for the population variance:

$$\sigma^2 = \frac{\sum_{i=1}^{N}(xi - \mu)^2}{N}$$

It seems complicated, but in fact it is not. It says that the population *variance* (σ^2) equals the sum of the difference of the population mean (μ) subtracted from all the data (xi) squared and then divided by the total population (N).

In most of the cases, it is not possible to calculate the population variance since we cannot obtain data from the entire population (i.e. every person in the world). Therefore, we need to calculate the sample variance:

$$S_{n-1}^2 = \frac{\sum_{i=1}^{n}(xi - \bar{x})^2}{n-1}$$

The above formula for sample variance is very similar to that for the population variance (σ^2); however, this time we use n (the sample population) as the denominator rather than N (the overall population).

In fact, when calculating the sample variance, we use $n - 1$ as the denominator because using just n would give us a biased estimate that significantly underestimates variability. Sample variance tends to be lower than real variance of the overall population. Reducing the population sample from n to $n - 1$ renders the variance intentionally large, providing an unbiased estimate of variability, taking into account that it is advised to overestimate rather than underestimate variability in samples.

Notably, we can't do the same with SD. Since SD is a square root and is not a linear operation, the procedure of subtraction (or addition) will not give the same unbiased calculation as the sample variance formula.

The SD (named also σ for the population) is calculated using the formula:

$$\sigma = \sqrt{\sigma^2}$$

For the sake of simplicity, it is the square root of variance. Let's work through a practical example where we consider the length of the post-operative stay (in days) of 6 patients who included the broccoli dietary regimen before heart surgery.

The dataset is 7, 12, 32, 10, 9 and 8. Each value represents the number of days of in-hospital stay of 6 patients after surgery. The mean ($\overline{x}$ with a "hat") is calculated to be:

$\overline{x} = (7+12+32+10+9+8)/6 = 13$

For the second step, we must subtract the mean ($\overline{x} = 13$) from each of the values of the 6 patients in order to calculate the deviation from the mean, as set out below:

Variable (days)	Mean ($\overline{x}$)	Deviation from the mean
7	13	7−13 = −6
12	13	12−13 = −1
32	13	32−13 = 19
10	13	10−13 = −3
9	13	9−13 = −4
8	13	8−13 = −5

Notably, some numbers are negative. To overcome this problem, our third step is to square each deviation from the mean as follows:

Squared deviation from the mean ($\overline{x}$)	
$(-6)^2$	36
$(-1)^2$	1
$(19)^2$	361
$(-3)^2$	9
$(-4)^2$	16
$(-5)^2$	25

Next, we must calculate the "sum of square": 36+1+361+9+16+25=448

Finally, we need to divide the sum of square by either $n - 1$ or N. Since we are working with a sample population of $n = 6$, we calculate $448/6 - 1$.

The sample variance is 448/5 = 89.6. The SD is 9.5 days (square root of the variance).

With this we can conclude that, in our experiment, the mean post-operative length of stay in the above sample of patients who included the dietary broccoli regimen was 13 ± 9.5 days, with a variance of 89.6.

Thankfully "R" calculates the variance for us if we build the new vector "length of stay" (LOS):

```
> LOS<-c(7,12,32,10,9,8)
> var(LOS)
[1] 89.6
```

It confirms our calculation.

Then, "R" can calculate the SD for us:

```
> sd(LOS)
[1] 9.46
```

6.7 Standard Error of the Mean vs Standard Deviation

We take a sample from a general population since we want to make inference about the latter. How similar to the general population is our sample? For instance, how much does the mean of our sample differ compared to the true mean of the general population? We can estimate how much the mean of the sampling distribution varies from the mean of the true population with the SE.

However, we need to make some clarification between variance, standard deviation and standard error.

The concept of the sample variance (s^2) and the standard deviation SD ($\sqrt{s^2}$) is specific. They represent the variability of the observations from the sample mean. Specifically, the sample variance and the SD quantify the variation within a set of measurements (e.g. our sample of interest set out above). The SE quantifies *the variation in the means from multiple sets of measurements*; in simple words *the SE is the standard deviation of the means*.

This might be confusing since the SE can be estimated just from a single set of measurements (even though it describes the means from multiple sets).

The SE ($\sigma_{\bar{x}}$) depends on the sample size and on the SD itself.

It is very important to remember that as the sample size increases, the SE decreases (i.e. a bigger sample size = higher precision). In contrast, increasing the sample size does not make the SD necessarily larger or smaller; it simply becomes a more accurate estimate of the population SD.

The SE formula is given below:

$$\text{SE} = \frac{\sigma}{\sqrt{n}}$$

where σ is the standard deviation and n is the sample size.

Below is the code required for "R" to calculate the SE of the sample10 object:

```
> std_mean <- function(sample10) sd(sample10)/sqrt(length(sample10))
```

However, in a scientific paper we rarely include the SE as a measure of precision of the sampling distribution, since we are more interested in the variability of the sample defined by the SD.

6.8 Accuracy and Confidence Intervals

We have discussed what precision means. The larger the sample size, the more precise our point of estimate (smaller standard error of the mean). But what is accuracy? To understand accuracy, we must discuss confidence intervals.

If 100 samples are taken and a 95% confidence interval (CI) is calculated, approximately 95 out of the 100 samples will contain the true population mean. Simply speaking, the CI is a range of values that is likely to include the population mean with a certain degree of confidence.

The accuracy is then defined in terms of whether or not the CI contains the true population parameter. As the confidence level increases (e.g., we set it from 95% to 99%), the width of the CI increases as well. Which then increases accuracy.

Considering the example dataset, we can foresee that patients after surgery will bleed between 1 mL and 2L of blood during the first 24 h. This is very likely and accurate, and such a wide range would certainly reflect the event. However, such a huge confidence level (high accuracy) is not very helpful and won't tell us how to clinically behave.

It means that the precision decreases. The precision in fact refers to the width of the CI.

More accuracy means a higher CI but with less precision. There is a trade-off between accuracy and precision. The only way to maximise both of them is to increase the sample size.

For a large sample, a 95% CI is obtained from the values 1.96×SE either side of the mean.

Let's create a practical example for the purpose of clarification. Using a study sample of $n = 50$, which contains patients who included the broccoli dietary regimen 1 week before surgery, the mean length of the post-operative stay was 14 days ± 2 (the latter indicates the SD). The SE from the (unknown) population mean would be:

$$SE = \frac{2}{\sqrt{50}} = \frac{2}{7.07} = 0.28$$

and the 95% CI would be 1.96 × 0.28 = 0.54, which means that the mean post-operative length of stay is 14 ± 2 and we are 95% confident that the true mean is somewhere between 14.28 and 13.72.

6.9 Mean, Median, Mode

Now to discuss the mean, median and mode. These are the most popular and known population and sample parameters and measures of central tendency.

We know that for the normal standard distribution, mean, median and mode are equivalent.

Before proceeding for summary and analysis, we should check for normality distribution, as set out in Chap. 5. When the sample n is normally distributed, we should use the mean along with the SD. We also know that for large samples we can assume normality (as per the central limit theory). When a sample is not normally distributed, we should then use the median and interquartile range.

How to check for normality both graphically and numerically was outlined in Chap. 5 (using the hypothesis test with the Shapiro test). Included was the use of boxplot. There was an analysis of the median. In the second boxplot Q2 represents the median, and Q1 − Q3 the interquartile range.

Once again, outliers play a pivotal role. Not surprisingly, the mean is heavily affected by outliers, while the median is not. Let's investigate why.

Referring to the arithmetic mean as per the formula below (probably one of the most known formulas in statistics):

$$\overline{X} = \frac{\sum_{i=1}^{n} X_i}{n} = \frac{x_1 + x_2 + \ldots x_n}{n}$$

This time we use the MMstat$LOS object and will apply the function mean (it seems we do not have many covariates normally distributed in our dataset):

```
> mean(MMstat$LOS)
[1] NA
```

In this case "R" is affected by the missing values in the columns of the covariate

`MMstat$LOS.`

We should prompt "R" to ignore them as below:

```
> mean(MMstat$LOS, na.rm=TRUE)
[1] 14.71
```

The function na.rm is very important since in the real world you will often have a lot of data missing from a dataset.

It is important to understand that there are many other types of mean, such as geometric, weighted, etc., which won't be described here.

It goes without saying that extreme values will affect the calculation of the mean, e.g. a small number of patients with complications, who remain in hospital for many weeks, will affect the mean. One possibility (in place of calculating the mean) is to trim values. To compute a trimmed mean, we remove a predetermined number of observations from each side of a distribution:

```
> mean(MMstat$LOS, na.rm=TRUE, trim=0.1)
[1] 13.23
```

and with the argument trim we are erasing a 0.1 fraction from each end of the distribution.

When trim=0.1 is used, 1 value from each end will be dropped from the calculation to find the trimmed mean.

Notably, the more you trim, the more you are excluding the outliers; therefore, the closer the mean gets to the median. Nevertheless, trimming may be a biased option, and it might instead be best to simply consider the median.

The median is the middle value, the 50th percentile. Fifty percent of the values are below the median, the other 50% above it. Median calculation is very easy, e.g. we create the vector:

```
> medianLOS<-c(2,4,5,11,4,5,78,3,4,5)
# sort the value in descending or ascending order
> sort(medianLOS, decreasing=FALSE)
 [1]  2  3  4  4  4  5  5  5 11 78
# find the central value, in this case the vector length is equal
to 10 (even number), hence we need to select the two central values
(4 and 5) and divide by 2.
> (4+5)/2
[1] 4.5
```

For confirmation we can use the function median:

```
> median(medianLOS)
[1] 4.5
```

The mode is the value that has the highest number of occurrences (frequencies) in a dataset. Unlike mean and median, mode can have both numeric and character data. Surprisingly, "R" does not have a standard built-in function to calculate the mode. We can create an ad hoc getmode function as below:

```
> getmode <- function(v) {
    uniqv <- unique(v)
    uniqv[which.max(tabulate(match(v, uniqv)))]
> getmode(MMstat$Age)
[1] 72
```

We now know that 72 years is the age most represented (has the highest frequency) in our dataset (the mode). The mode can also be used for non-numeric variables. Let's use diabetes as an example. It has three levels (0, 1, 2). Which is the most represented? The mode will tell us:

```
> getmode(MMstat$Diabetes)
[1] 0
```

Also, for categorical variables, you can use the table function:

```
> table(MMstat$Diabetes)
  0   1   2
413  71  16
```

The table function for categorical variables tells us not only the highest frequency but also the exact frequency of each value.

The summary function can also be helpful. It returns the minimum and maximum values, the 1st and 3rd quartiles, the median and the mean.

```
> summary(MMstat$Height)
   Min. 1st Qu.  Median    Mean 3rd Qu.    Max.
  146.0   160.0   166.0   167.4   174.0   196.0
```

6.10 Conclusion

Small samples will lead to little accuracy and precision. While the standard error of the mean tells us how precise our sample (n) is compared to the population (N), sample variance and standard deviation are measures of variability of the sample observations around the sample mean.

In biostatistics, if the sample is large enough and normally distributed, we report numbers as mean and standard deviation. Otherwise, median and interquartile range are used. In scientific papers, the standard error of the mean is rarely considered. Additionally, the standard deviation is preferred over the variance. The 95% confidence interval is the most frequent confidence level used in biostatistics. It says that we are 95% confident the true mean is within a range. It also tells us about the amount of information: the more data, the shorter the confidence interval.

Further Readings

Dawson B, Trapp RG. Basic and clinical biostatistics. 4th ed. New York: McGraw Hill; 2004.

Manikandan S. Measures of central tendency: median and mode. J Pharmacol Pharmacother. 2011;2:214–5.

McLeod SA. What are confidence intervals in statistics? Simply psychology; 2019, June 10. Available from: https://www.simplypsychology.org/confidence-interval.html

Norman GR, Streiner DL. Biostatistics the bare essentials. 2nd ed. Hamilton: B.C. Decker Inc; 2000.

Chapter 7
Correlation

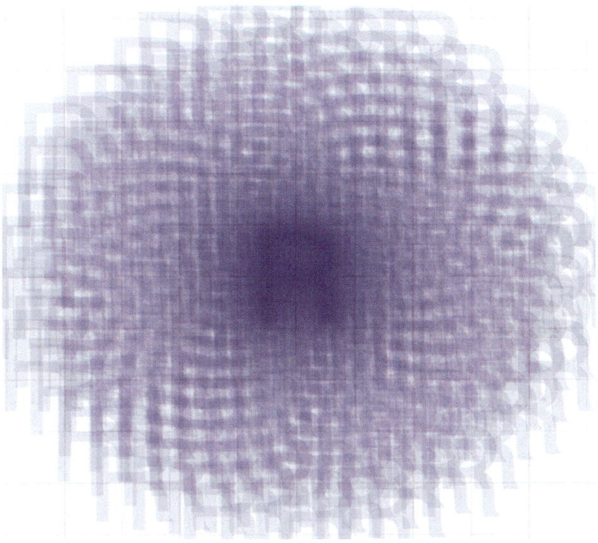

7.1 Software and R-Packages Required for This Chapter

If you haven't already, you need to download and install base-R and R-studio as set out in Chap. 2 under the heading "Downloading "R" and R-studio".

M. Moscarelli, *Biostatistics With 'R': A Guide for Medical Doctors*, https://doi.org/10.1007/978-3-031-33073-5_7

The relevant R-packages needed for this chapter are:

- tidyverse—it can be downloaded at: http://tidyverse.tidyverse.org
- corrplot—it can be downloaded at: https://github.com/taiyun/corrplot
- ggcorrplot—it can be downloaded at: http://www.sthda.com/english/wiki/ggcorrplot

7.2 Where to Download the Example Dataset and the Script for This Chapter

If you haven't already downloaded the supplementary dataset named `MMstat.csv` created as a practical example for use throughout this book, you will find it at the link that follows. The script for this chapter named `Chapter 7.Correlation.R` can also be found and downloaded at the following link:

https://github.com/mmlondon77/Biobook.git

7.3 What Is Correlation?

Two numeric covariates may show a certain relationship (correlation) when they "move" towards the same direction (positive correlation) or in opposite directions (negative correlation). However, you have probably heard the famous statement "correlation does not mean causation". A set of only two variables may not be sufficient to build a statistical model which infers x is linked to y, when there is the possibility that another variable z exists and z is in fact the real cause of y.

Sadly, correlation can only be measured between two variables at a time.

Correlation is often considered a part of descriptive statistics and can be positive, negative, no correlation (flat line), linear and non-linear.

A correlation not significantly different from 0 means that there is no linear relationship between the two variables considered. However, there could be another non-linear association.

This chapter will mainly cover the Pearson's method as a measure of quantifying the *magnitude* and *direction* of correlation. Correlation goes from -1 (*perfect negative* correlation) to $+1$ (*perfect positive* correlation) where 0 indicates no correlation.

There are other correlation coefficients, such as *Kendall* or *Spearman*, but the most used is *Pearson*. We will also briefly examine Spearman, which is the non-parametric version of Pearson. You will in fact see that Pearson's correlation coefficient is based on assumptions that must hold, including linearity between the two variables in analysis.

7.4 Correlation Plots

The figure below contains two correlation plots (Fig. 7.1):

The plot on the left shows *positive* correlation between the *x* and *y* variables. High *x* measurements correspond to high *y* measurements. Therefore, when *x* variables increase, so do *y* variables (i.e. *x* and *y* move towards the same direction). Vice versa the plot on the right shows *negative* correlation. As *x* increases, *y* tends to decrease (i.e. *x* and *y* move in opposite directions).

We can make many examples of positive correlation, such as height and weight (taller people tend to be heavier) or time spent on the treadmill and calories burnt, atmospheric temperature and ice cream sales. There are some examples of negative correlation, such as car speed and travel time, atmospheric temperature and hot drink sales.

Notably, plotting data always helps you understand the direction and perhaps the magnitude of the relationship between two continuous variables.

If the correlation coefficient between two variables is close to or at zero, the plot would look similar to the one below (Fig. 7.2):

The two variables *x* and *y* seem unrelated with no relationship. The grey line (called best fit regression line) is almost flat. However, we may just conclude that there is no linear relationship, but some other kind of non-linear relationship might apply to the model.

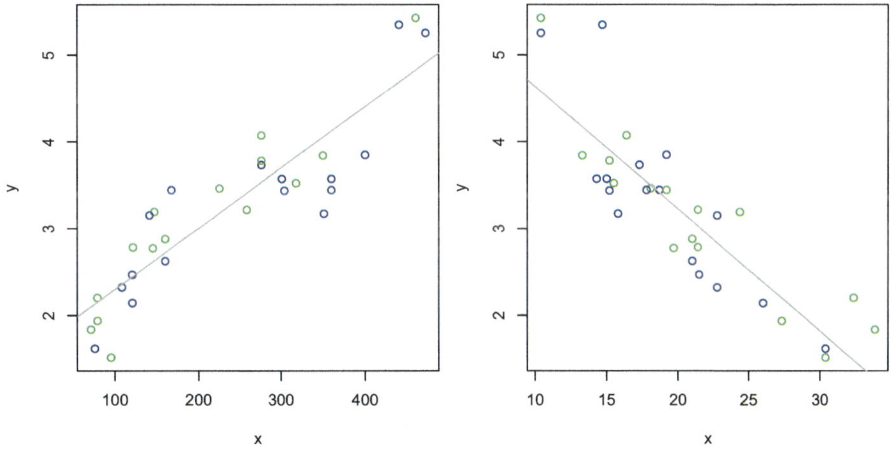

Fig. 7.1 Positive correlation (left) and negative correlation (right)

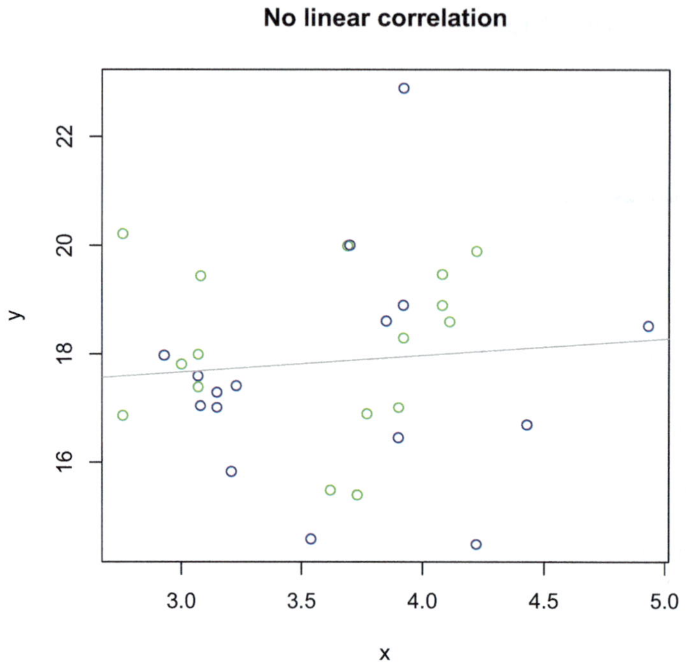

Fig. 7.2 No significant correlation between *x* and *y* variables

7.5 Exploring Correlation Using the Example Dataset

Our example dataset `MMstat` contains some numeric continuous variables, such as height, weight, creatinine, bleeding, etc. We can check the structure of these variables with the function `str( )`.

Some of the patients' baseline characteristics or perioperative variables may have an effect on post-operative bleeding. For instance, we may hypothesise that patients with renal dysfunction, causing higher creatinine levels, may have a higher tendency of post-operative bleeding. Longer operation time and ischaemic time may also correlate to post-operative bleeding.

We can start exploring potential relationships between cross-clamp/ischaemic time and bleeding, using the following code (Fig. 7.3):

```
>    plot(MMstat$Bleeding~MMstat$CC,     col=c('blue',     'green'),
xlab='Cross clamp or ischemic time min', ylab='Bleeding ml')
> abline(lm(MMstat$Bleeding~MMstat$CC), col="red")
```

In general, statistical practice, variables which are the outcome of interest, in this case the post-operative bleeding, are plotted on the *y*-axis, while the variables that may affect the outcome of interest, in this case the cross-clamp/ischaemic time, are

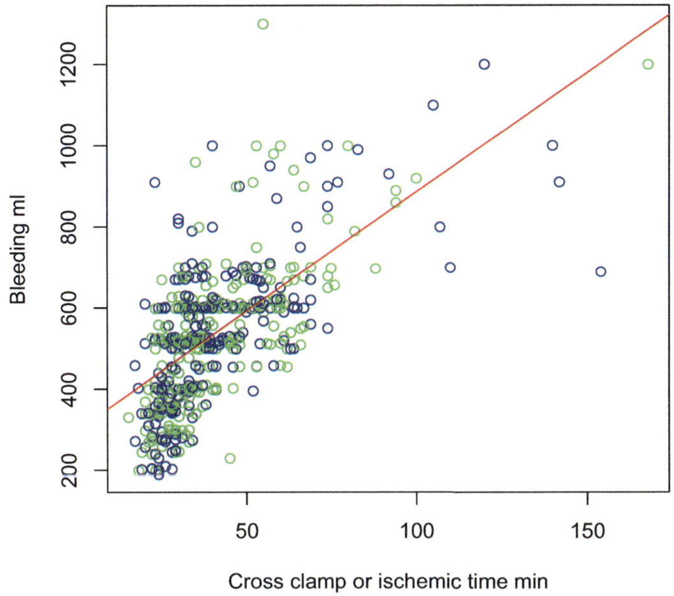

Fig. 7.3 Correlation plot

plotted on the *x*-axis. The outcome of interest is also called the *dependent variable*, since it can be affected by other variables. The variable which may affect the dependent variable is named the *independent variable*. You will see why such nomenclature is helpful when we examine regression.

In order to depict the two variables (dependent `Bleeding` variable = y-axis, and independent `CC` variable = x-axis), we use the function `plot( )`. After parenthesis I should include the outcome of interest (`Bleeding`) followed by the variable that may affect it (`CC`). The symbol ~ (tilde), which you will often see in regression, says that the dependent variable is affected by the independent variable. The rest of the code is intuitive: colours are assigned at the two variables `col=c('blue', 'green')`, and afterwards the *x*- and *y*-axes are named `xlab='Cross clamp or ischemic time min', ylab='Bleeding ml'`.

In the second code, the `abline( )` function is introduced (for the regression line/the line of best fit). Notably, this is the line that best expresses the relationship between those points in the scatterplot and may give a sense of the direction and magnitude of the relationship between the two variables. This is covered in more depth later in the book about linear regression. For the time being, you can see how the linear model `lm( )` function is entered to build and plot the regression line above. The linear model function is used to visualise and understand better the effect of `CC` on `Bleeding`, after plotting the dependent variable `Bleeding` against `CC` (i.e. I need to understand how `CC` (x) affects post-operative `Bleeding` (y)).

7.6 Interpretation of the Correlation Scatterplot

Scatterplot means the values are scattered across the plot. We scatter observations from only two variables at a time, in this example `Bleeding` (*y*-axis) and `CC` (*x*-axis). It may be intuitive that a positive relationship/correlation between those two variables exists, and as the x-axis values increase, so do the y-axis values.

But how strong is this positive relationship? Is it significant? To understand that we can use the function `cor.test( )`:

```
> cor.test(MMstat$Bleeding, MMstat$CC, method='pearson')
   Pearson's product-moment correlation
data:  MMstat$Bleeding and MMstat$CC
t = 18.633, df = 498, p-value < 0.01
alternative hypothesis: true correlation is not equal to 0
95 % confidence interval:0.58 0.68
sample estimates: cor 0.64
```

As you can see above, highlighted in red shows the correlation is positive at 0.64 (being between 0 for no linear correlation and 1 for maximum correlation) and the p-value is significant ($p < 0.01$). We can conclude that `Bleeding` and `CC` have a positive/significant relationship, as `CC` increases, `Bleeding` increases.

The variables have a positive correlation of 0.64, but does it mean that `CC` causes `Bleeding`? We cannot draw such a conclusion. As outlined earlier correlation does not mean causation. A more complex statistical model should be constructed to answer this research question.

7.7 Pearson's Correlation

For the example above, Pearson's correlation was used. Pearson's correlation is a measure of the strength of a *linear* association between two continuous variables.

It must be emphasised that, in order to use Pearson's method, the behaviour of two variables must be linear.

In fact, in order to use Pearson's correlation, several necessary conditions must be satisfied:

i.) Both variables are continuous.
ii.) Observations are a random sample from the population.
iii.) Both variables are approximately normally distributed within the population.
iv.) Most importantly, the relationship between the two variables is linear.

Please consider that Pearson's correlation is extremely sensitive to sample size and a small population may return misleading statistical information.

The statistic associated with Pearson's correlation is reported with the letter *r*. As a rule of thumb, the association can be weak, moderate or strong, besides no correlation at all or theoretically perfect correlation.

r	Strength of association
±0.7	Strong correlation
±0.5	Moderate correlation
±0.3	Weak correlation
±0.0	No correlation

Taking into consideration the assumptions listed above (linearity and normality of the random samples), it might not be right to use Pearson's correlation coefficient. If we look at the scatterplot `Bleeding / CC`, the linearity assumption may not hold. Also, both variables, dependent and independent, do not look normally distributed.

7.8 Is This Correlation Linear?

We have assumed that the relationship between `Bleeding` (dependent variable *y*-axis) and `CC` (independent variable *x*-axis) is linear. However, if we use `ggplot`, we visualise a smoothed regression line which indicates the linearity assumption will not hold; see below (Fig. 7.4):

```
> ggplot(MMstat, aes(x=CC, y=Bleeding)) + geom_point()+ geom_smooth()
```

Also, both dependent and independent variables are not normally distributed. This may suggest that outliers affect the model. Scattering is a good way to detect abnormal observations (see the right side of the above plot) or a gap in the distribution.

Data may require some transformation for further analysis. You will see that this is particularly true for linear regression analysis.

For this, we should explore `log( )` transformation which is easily performed in "R" (Fig. 7.5):

```
>     plot(log(MMstat$Bleeding)~log(MMstat$CC),      col=c('blue',
'green'), xlab='log CC time', ylab='log Bleeding')
> abline(lm(log(MMstat$Bleeding)~log(MMstat$CC), col="red"))
```

Interestingly, the correlation is now more linear after log transformation. Nevertheless, the vast majority of relationships in regression statistics can be described on the basis of linearity. We will discuss linearity and non-linearity more on regression.

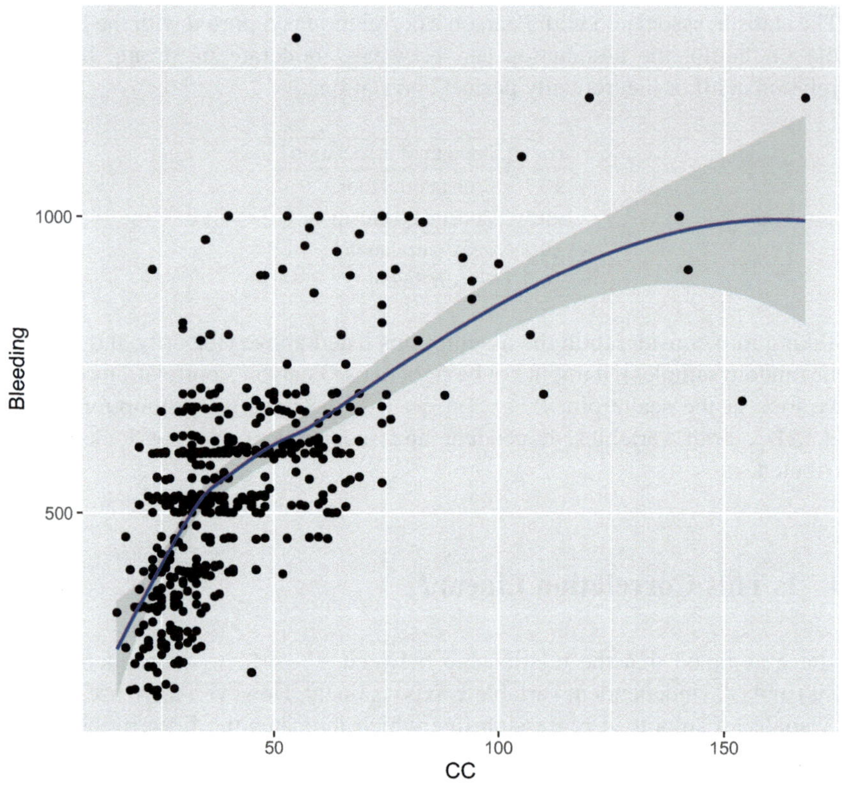

Fig. 7.4 Visualising smoothed relationship between cc and bleeding

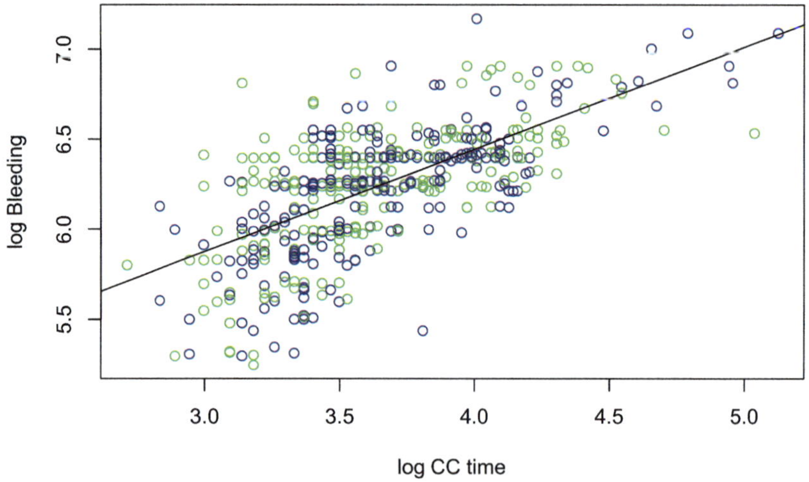

Fig. 7.5 Scatterplot after log transformation

7.9 Spearman's Correlation

Spearman's correlation coefficient is the non-parametric version of Pearson's correlation coefficient. As a reminder, non-parametric means we do not make any assumptions around the form of the data; hence, we do not assume it follows a specific distribution (i.e. normal distribution).

Conversely to Pearson's correlation, Spearman does not require distributional assumptions about the variables. This may be useful for our variables `Bleeding` and `CC`, which are not normally distributed.

However, Spearman requires that there be a *monotonic* relationship between variables; in a monotonic relationship, the variables tend to move towards the same direction but not at constant rate (contrary to linear relation).

Spearman's statistics has less restriction than Pearson. However, even in this scenario, some conditions must hold:

i.) There is a monotonic relationship between the two variables.
ii.) Both variables should be either continuous or ordinal.
iii.) Observations must come from a random sample of the population.

Let's try to calculate the Spearman's correlation with the code below:

```
> cor(MMstat$Bleeding, MMstat$CC, method = 'spearman')

[1] 0.63
```

You will see I changed the specification `method = 'spearman'`; notably the strength of the association is very similar in this case to the Pearson's coefficient:

```
> cor(MMstat$Bleeding, MMstat$CC, method = 'pearson')
[1] 0.64
```

7.10 Correlation Matrix

As outlined before, correlation can only be measured and plotted between two variables at a time. In previous paragraphs we investigate the relationship between two variables from the example dataset `MMstat`. Our variable of interest is the bleeding covariate, which records the amount of post-operative bleeding (measured in mL), and a possible cause for it, the cross-clamp or ischaemic time `CC`. Both of them are numeric variables. However, our dataset has many numeric variables that theoretically may have a relationship (can correlate) with our outcome of interest. Computing correlation for each of them and performing plotting can be time and space consuming. A practical solution to this problem would be to use a matrix system (such as *correlation matrix*), which shows correlation direction, coefficient (and potentially p-value) for all possible combinations of two variables in a dataset.

We have previously learnt that we can subset the dataset using either the basic "R" function (in squared brackets `[ ]`) or we can use the `dplyr` function from the `tidyverse` R-package.

Let's start with the basic "R" function for data wrangling, to select only the columns with continuous numeric data and create an object named `MMnumeric` (a subset which contains only continuous variables from the dataset):

```
> MMnumeric<-MMstat[,c(2,4,5,8,9,12,13,14,16)]#numbers indicate
the columns which contain numeric variables
```

Remember you can always use the `View( )` function to visualise the object `MMnumeric`.

We can then use the function `cor` and choose to round to two decimals as below (Fig. 7.6):

```
> round(cor(MMnumeric), 2)
```

Here I have created a correlation matrix of all continuous variables from the dataset. As highlighted in red, the correlation coefficient (using Pearson) between `Bleeding` and `CC` is 0.64, which suggests there is a positive correlation between the two variables as strong as 0.64 (1 being the *perfect* or maximum positive correlation). Note that there are `NAs` in the matrix since the `LOS` variable contains missing values. Note also that, for the sake of simplicity, we calculate it using Pearson's coefficient, yet linearity may not hold.

Nevertheless, you may agree with me that the matrix reported above may not be easily and quickly interpretable. It would be better to plot all correlation coefficients at once. We do that with the following code (Fig. 7.7):

```
> round(cor(MMnumeric), 2)
             Age Weight Height  LVEF Creatinine   CPB    CC LOS Bleeding
Age         1.00  -0.08  -0.29 -0.01       0.22 -0.07 -0.18  NA    -0.07
Weight     -0.08   1.00   0.47  0.02       0.17  0.10  0.11  NA     0.09
Height     -0.29   0.47   1.00 -0.04       0.21  0.16  0.17  NA     0.16
LVEF       -0.01   0.02  -0.04  1.00       0.01 -0.07  0.00  NA    -0.05
Creatinine  0.22   0.17   0.21  0.01       1.00  0.13  0.13  NA     0.11
CPB        -0.07   0.10   0.16 -0.07       0.13  1.00  0.72  NA     0.85
CC         -0.18   0.11   0.17  0.00       0.13  0.72  1.00  NA     0.64
LOS           NA     NA     NA    NA         NA    NA    NA   1       NA
Bleeding   -0.07   0.09   0.16 -0.05       0.11  0.85  0.64  NA     1.00
```

Fig. 7.6 Correlation matrix

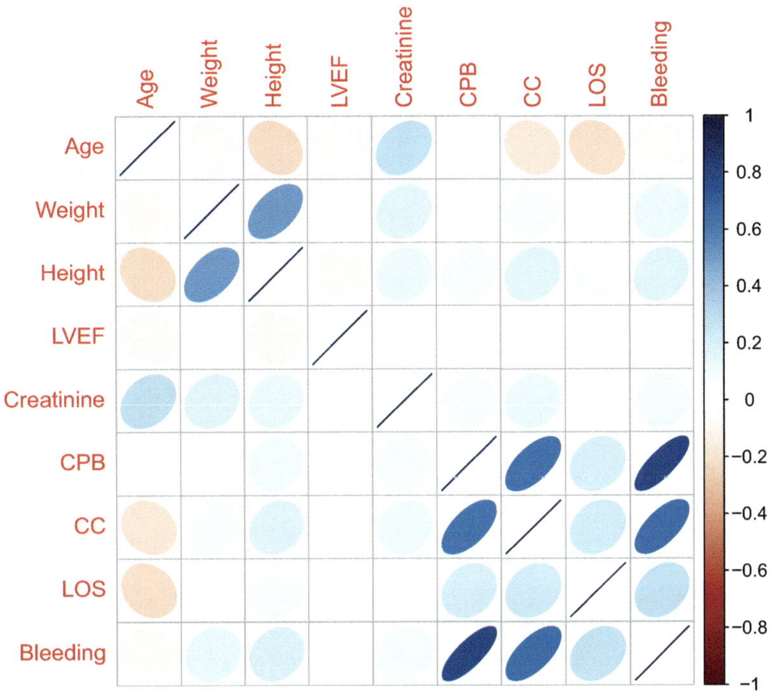

Fig. 7.7 Correlation matrix with corrplot (method="ellipse")

```
> library(corrplot)
> pairs(MMnumeric, col="darkgreen")
> mycor<-(cor(MMnumeric))
> corrplot(mycor, method="ellipse", na.label = 'NA')
```

Note I use the argument `na.label = 'NA'` in order to remove the missing observations from the `LOS` covariate. Also, positive correlations are displayed in blue and negative correlations in red. I use the argument `method="ellipse"` whereby the sharper the ellipse, the stronger the correlation (i.e. the closer to either -1 or 1) and which also intensifies the colour proportional to the strength of the correlation coefficient (i.e. the stronger the correlation, the darker the colour). The colour legend on the right-hand side of the matrix depicts the correlation coefficients and the corresponding colours.

We may want to instead add the coefficient numbers into the plot; we do this by changing the `method` argument as below (Fig. 7.8):

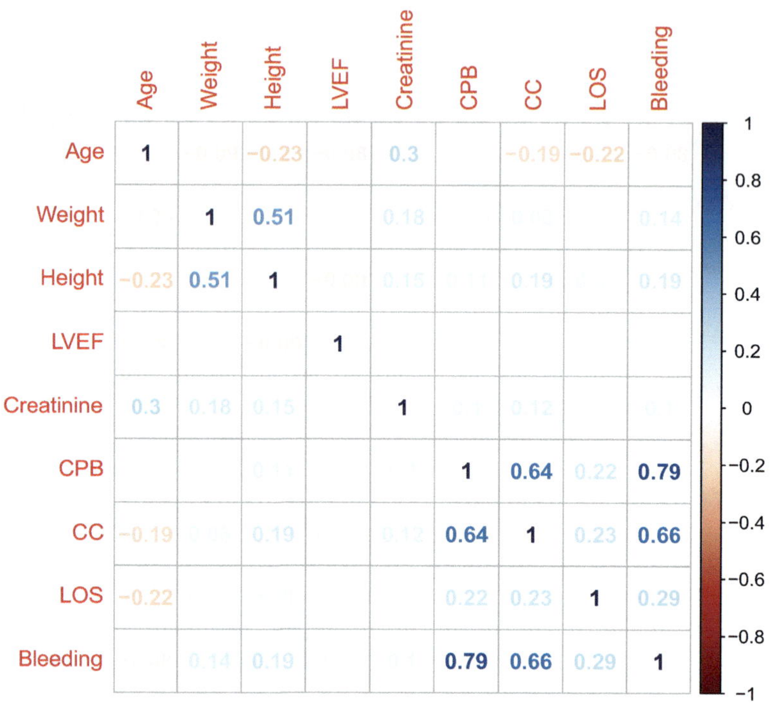

Fig. 7.8. Correlation matrix with correlation coefficients

```
> corrplot(mycor, method=c( 'number'))
```

7.11 Are Correlation Coefficients Important?

Correlation coefficients tell us about the direction of relationships between two variables (continuous variables only) and the strength of the relationships. Nothing more, nothing less. Correlation is a process that is part of descriptive statistics and may help us in trying to understand what research question to conceive. From the correlation matrix above, I can make out that both `CPB` and `CC` have a positive correlation with `Bleeding` (0.79 and 0.66, respectively). Do they cause bleeding? In order to answer this question, we must build a more complex statistical model, not just bivariate ($y \sim x$) rather a multivariable model ($y \sim x + z \ldots$), which takes into account many covariates that may be of interest because they may contribute to post-operative bleeding. Why can't we blindly rely on correlations? One of the most famous examples is the correlation between shark attacks and ice cream sales. If we consider those two variables *uncritically*, we will probably find that indeed there is a positive correlation between the two. Anytime ice cream sales increase, the number of shark attacks increase. However, the obvious explanation is that a third omitted variable *atmospheric temperature* is the real cause of the increase in shark attacks, because in summer people swim more. We should always consider that perhaps omitted variables from a statistical model (in this case *atmospheric temperature*) are in fact pivotal. Going back to our dataset, the question whether CC or CPB cause bleeding can only be answered if we include them in a more complex and comprehensive model. This model is called *regression model* and will be covered in its dedicated chapter later in the book.

7.12 Elegant Correlation Matrices

I now demonstrate using the ggplot2 package to produce the same scatterplots. While before I used the basic functionality for subsetting to select only continuous variables, this section shows you how to do the same using the dplyr library from the tidyverse R-package:

```
# library(dplyr)
> MMnumeric <- MMstat %>%
  dplyr::select_if(is.numeric)
> mycor<-(cor(MMnumeric))
```

Note that %>% is commonly used as an operator in the dplyr function. It can be used to chain code together, and it is very useful when you are performing several operations on data and don't want to save the output at each intermediate step. We can now use the ggcorrplot package and recall the mycor object previously created (Fig. 7.9):

```
> install.packages("ggcorrplot")
library(ggcorrplot)
ggcorrplot(mycor, method = "circle")

> ggcorrplot(mycor, type = "lower", lab = TRUE)
```

(Fig. 7.10)

The correlation matrix is similar to the one produced with basic graphic but probably neater. The type = "lower" coding displays the correlation matrix as a triangle in the lower part of the plot.

Lastly, we can produce a plot as set out below with the code (Fig. 7.11):

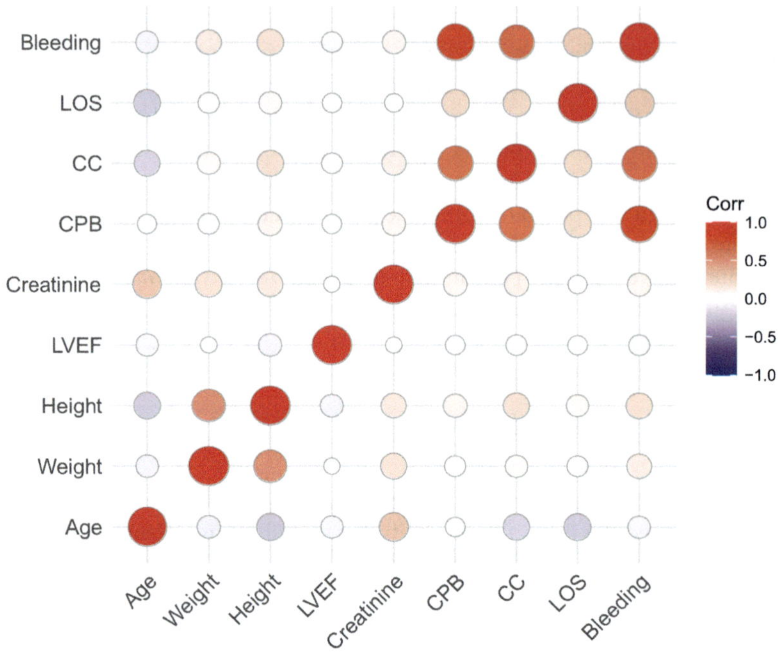

Fig. 7.9. Correlation matrix with ggcorrplot (method = "circle")

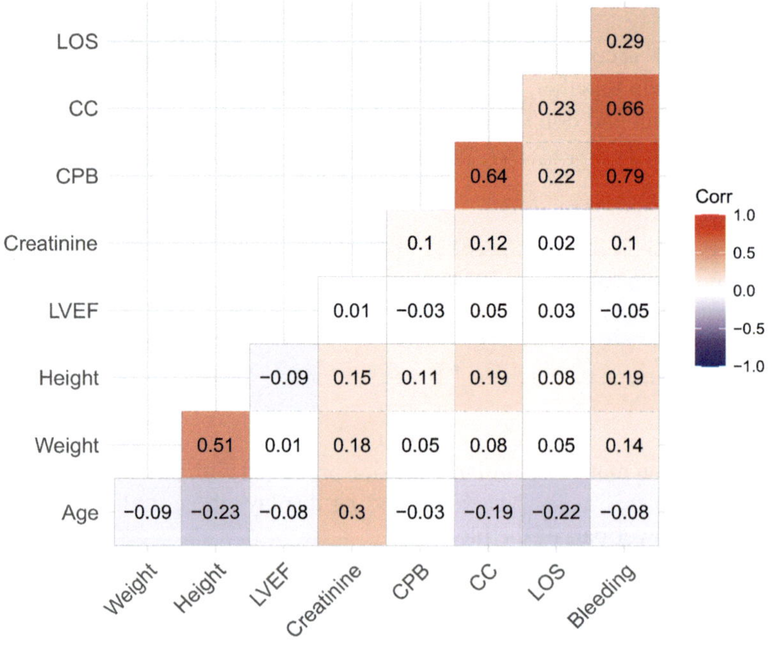

Fig. 7.10 Correlation matrix with ggcorrplot (type = "lower")

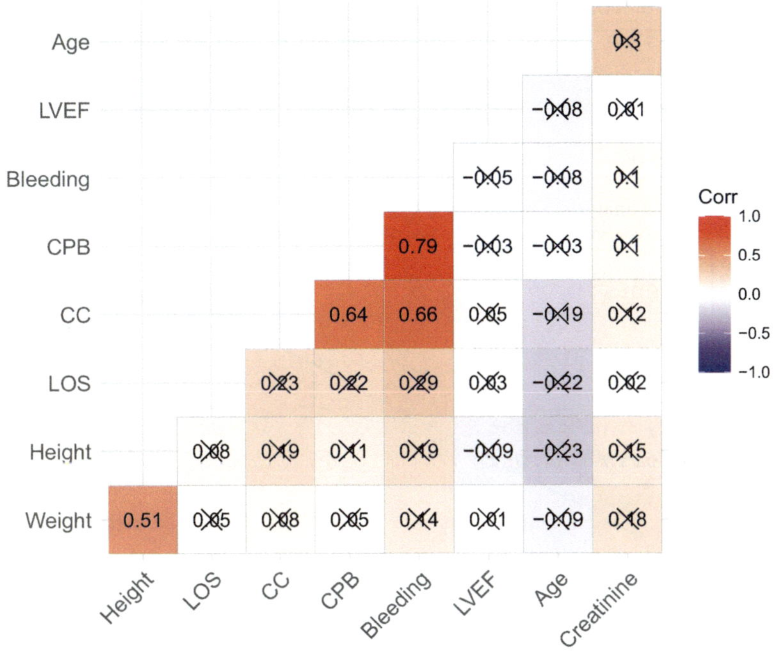

Fig. 7.11 Correlation matrix (with cor_pmat) with not significant correlations erased

```
> p.mat<-cor_pmat(mycor)
> ggcorrplot(mycor, hc.order=TRUE, type = "lower", lab = TRUE,
p.mat=p.mat)
```

The not significant correlations are erased with crosses. It is important to note `cor_pmat( )` returns a matrix containing the p-values of correlations. You might notice that our `Bleeding` outcome of interest correlates (significantly) with `CC` and `CPB`. Those two variables must definitely be included in a multivariable model!

7.13 Correlation with Two Intercepts (Stratified by Two Groups)

We should not lose sight of our original research question: “does the broccoli dietary regimen reduce post-operative bleeding?”

So far in this chapter, we have tried to answer the question of whether `CC` influences `Bleeding`, with regard to the overall population (whole cohort, *Broccoli* and *noBroccoli*). It is worthwhile to now delve deeper to try to understand, at least from a speculative point of view, the relationship between `Bleeding` and `CC`

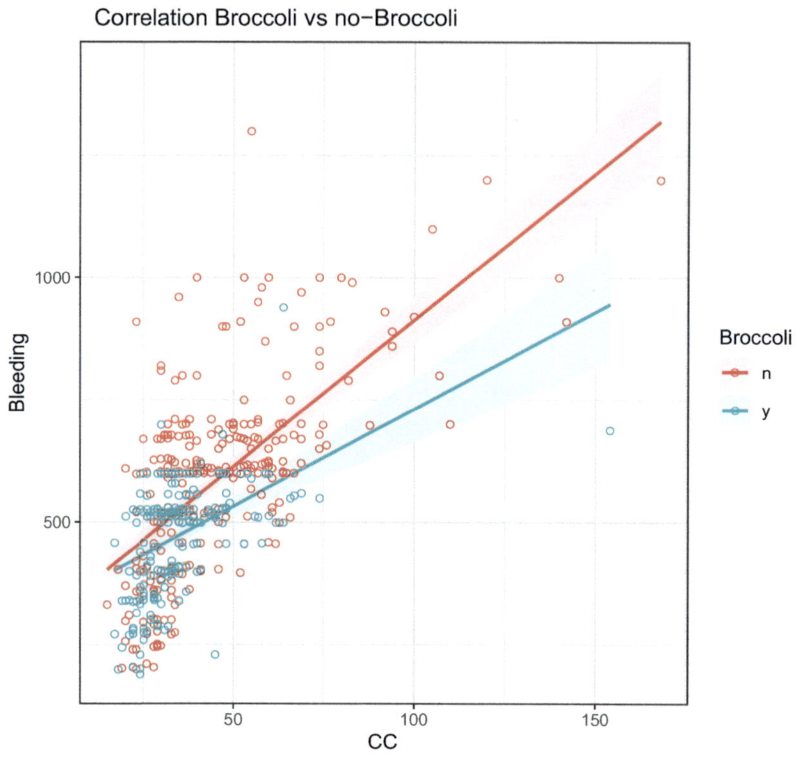

Fig. 7.12 Correlation plot grouped by Broccoli variable (*y*/*n*)

within each of the two groups of interest. Basically, does the relationship between `CC` and `Bleeding` differ according to the dietary regimen?

Once again, in order to answer this question, we use functions that belong to the `ggplot2` R-package (Fig. 7.12):

```
> ggplot(MMstat, aes(x=CC, y=Bleeding, color=Broccoli,
fill=Broccoli)) + geom_point(shape=1)+ geom_smooth(method = 'lm',
alpha=0.1)+theme_bw()+labs(y='Bleeding',
x='CC',title='Correlation')
```

There are some differences. Each group has a different relationship with `Bleeding`. It seems the slope in the group who included `Broccoli` before surgery is less steep, indicating a looser positive correlation. This is theoretically in line with our hypothesis; in fact we thought that broccoli, with its anti-inflammatory properties, may lower `Bleeding`. In essence these scatterplots are supporting our hypothesis, for the moment. How many variables does this scatterplot have? Two continuous variables. However, we have introduced a new categorical variable (the

`Broccoli` variable) since we have stratified the correlation according to the group. The plot is now more informative.

Let's consider intercepts. What is an intercept? For the moment I define an intercept as the y-value where the regression line (line of best fit) crosses the y-axis. Since here we have two regression lines, one for Broccoli and the other for noBroccoli, we have two intercepts.

Below I explain the code to obtain the two intercept scatterplots and, as I have done previously, break it down into layers:

```
> ggplot(MMstat, [prompts ggplot to use the dataset MMstat] aes(x=CC, y=Bleeding, color=Broccoli, fill=Broccoli)) + [codes for the x and y axes to represent the two variables of interest, the independent CC variable and the dependent Bleeding variable] geom_point(shape=1)+ [sets out for observations to be plotted as points, in this example shape=1 is used, however there are many possible shapes available] geom_smooth(method = 'lm', alpha=0.1) [is the smoothing function (note lm method is used for a straight line) then shading is added with alpha] +theme_bw() [selects a black and white theme] +labs(y='Bleeding', x='CC',title='Correlation') [names the x and y axes and creates the plot title].
```

The correlation can also be plotted separately by groups in two different windows (side-by-side plot) with the function `facet_grid( )`, and this time without `lm` method which now displays curved lines of best fit (Fig. 7.13):

```
>ggplot(MMstat, aes(x=CC, y=Bleeding, color=Broccoli, fill=Broccoli)) + geom_point(shape=1)+ geom_smooth(col='grey')+theme_bw()+labs(y='Bleeding', x='CC',title='Correlation / facet')+facet_grid(~Broccoli)
```

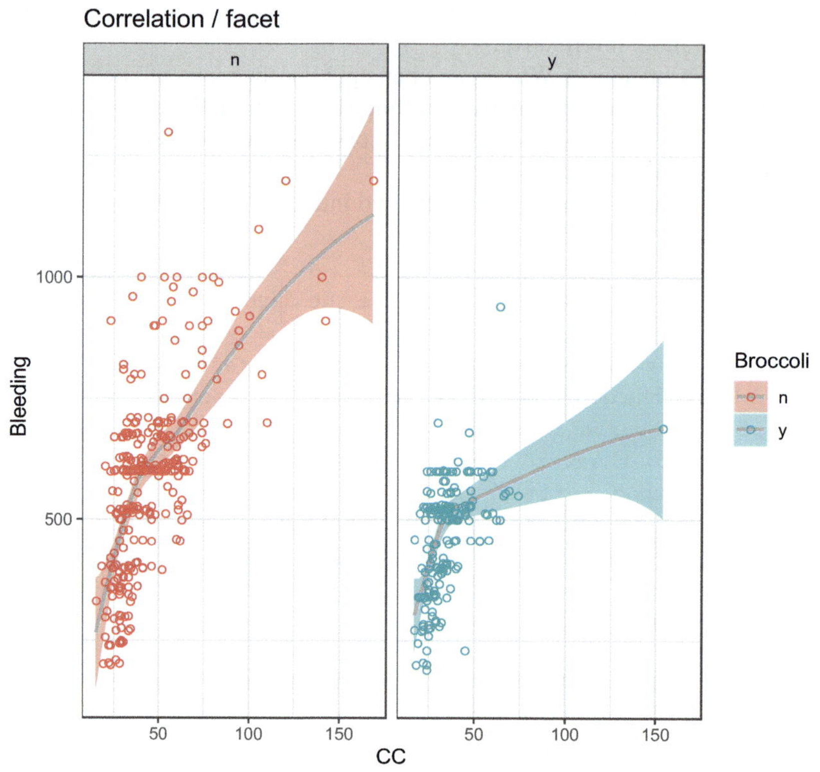

Fig. 7.13 Correlation grouped by Broccoli with a side-by-side plot (facet_grid) and curved lines of best fit

7.14 Conclusion

Correlation measures the strength of the association between two and only two variables. Correlation is often considered a part of descriptive statistics and can be positive, negative, no correlation (flat line), linear and non-linear. The most common form of correlation is between two numeric variables. By plotting the observations of the two variables on the *x*- and *y*-axes, we can highlight many characteristics of the variables themselves. It helps to understand if there is linearity between two variables, or where there are outliers or gaps in the distribution.

When the numeric variables come from a random sample and are normally distributed with linear behaviour, Pearson's correlation coefficient *r* can be computed. The value ranges from −1 (perfect negative correlation) to 1 (perfect positive correlation), whereby 0 indicates no correlation. A less restrictive form of Pearson is a non-parametric version, known as Spearman.

Correlations indicate magnitude and direction of two variables. For instance, considering the example dataset, we can establish that the longer the operation time during surgery (known as ischaemic time), the more the bleeding after surgery. However, I should again emphasise that correlation does not implicate causation, and in order to understand whether the ischaemic time might cause bleeding, a more complex model should be considered. What is then the value of correlation? Correlation analysis may give us more hints on what variables to include in a more advanced model (i.e. regression), and as such should be used as part of the descriptive or exploratory analysis.

Further Readings

Brace RA. Fitting straight lines to experimental data. Am J Physiol. 1977;233(3):R94–9. https://doi.org/10.1152/ajpregu.1977.233.3.R94.

Gaddis ML, Gaddis GM. Introduction to biostatistics: part 6, Correlation and regression. Ann Emerg Med. 1990;19(12):1462–8. https://doi.org/10.1016/s0196-0644(05)82622-8.

Kirch W, editor. Pearson's correlation coefficient. In: Encyclopedia of public health. Dordrecht: Springer; 2008. https://doi.org/10.1007/978-1-4020-5614-7_2569.

Rigby AS. Statistical methods in epidemiology. VI. Correlation and regression: the same or different? Disabil Rehabil. 2000;22(18):813–9. https://doi.org/10.1080/09638280050207857.

Schober P, Boer C, Schwarte LA. Correlation coefficients: appropriate use and interpretation. Anesth Analg. 2018;126(5):1763–8. https://doi.org/10.1213/ANE.0000000000002864.

Chapter 8
Hypothesis Testing

8.1 Software and R-Packages Required for This Chapter

If you haven't already, you need to download and install base-R and R-studio as set out in Chap. 2 under the heading "Downloading "R" and R-studio".

M. Moscarelli, *Biostatistics With 'R': A Guide for Medical Doctors*,
https://doi.org/10.1007/978-3-031-33073-5_8

The relevant R-package needed for this chapter is:

- tidyverse—it can be downloaded at http://tidyverse.tidyverse.org.

8.2 Where to Download the Example Dataset and Script for This Chapter

If you haven't already downloaded the supplementary dataset named `MMstat.csv` created as a practical example for use throughout this book, you will find it at the link that follows. The script for this chapter named `Chapter 8. Hypothesis testing.R` can also be found and downloaded at the following link:

https://github.com/mmlondon77/Biobook.git.

8.3 Fundamentals of Hypothesis Testing

In statistics, the null hypothesis (H_o) represents the *status quo*, the current belief of the parameter value. The *null* is also called the established value of the population parameter and is assumed to be true until we have very strong evidence to the contrary. For example, my null hypothesis could be the statement: "the earth is round". But before I demonstrate the contrary "the earth is flat" (the alternative hypothesis), I should have very solid evidence.

The alternative hypothesis (also named H_a or H_1) represents the challenge to the current belief about the population parameter value. The earth remains round *unless plausible evidence of the earth being flat is provided.* If I do not provide solid evidence to contrast the belief that the earth is round, I must *fail to reject the null hypothesis*. If I was to provide solid evidence of the earth being flat, I can *reject the null hypothesis*.

We have discussed descriptive and inferential statistics previously in this book. Hypothesis testing is a method of statistical inference.

H_o and H_a always come in a pair and are mathematical opposites. The earth is either round or flat. It cannot be both.

8.4 Probability Distribution

Hypothesis testing is based on probability distribution. In this chapter, this book covers the two most common: the normal distribution (Z) and the t-distribution, also named Student's t-distribution (t). In reality we may always use the latter t since the standard deviation from the general population is generally unknown; t is also indicated when we work with small sample sizes.

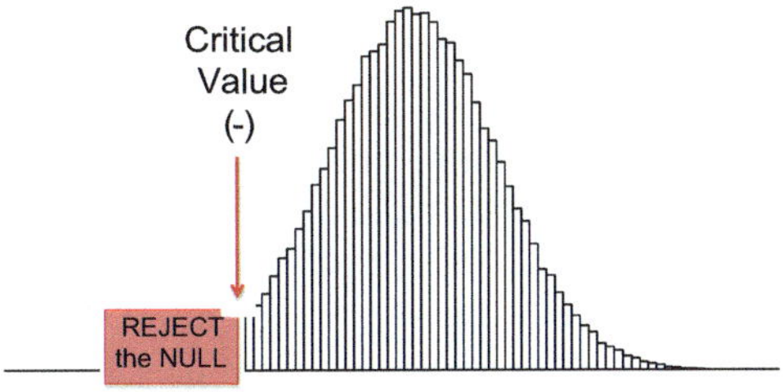

Fig. 8.1 Normal distribution with left rejection area. A critical value is a number or point on a test distribution that we compare to the test statistic to determine whether or not to reject the null hypothesis

T is a bell-curve-shaped distribution, approximately normally distributed, but with a lower peak and more observations at the level of the tails. This implies that we have higher probabilities to the tails than the normal standard distribution.

It is important to understand that we need probability distribution to locate the parameter of our sample of interest, e.g. if the average `Bleeding` (mL) of my sample falls towards the tails, either right or left (*rejection area*), far from the centre of *t* (*no-rejection area*), this value may be significant. You will see that the number that divides the rejection area (the tail) from the non-rejection area is named the *critical value*. We will discuss this value soon in this chapter.

I draw the figure below for a quick visual representation. It represents a normal distribution, with an area of rejection on the left. If the observation and the associated statistical test fall in this area of rejection, they unlikely represent the general population, so we acknowledge them as *significantly different* (Fig. 8.1).

It is clear we need probability distribution to perform hypothesis testing.

8.5 Normal and *t*-Distribution

Taking the example dataset into consideration, we conduct a study which investigates the effect of `Broccoli` on post-operative `Bleeding`, whereby we must compare the mean of the `Bleeding` variable from two groups. We start by calculating the mean from the collected data of post-operative `Bleeding` from the two populations expressed in mL. But in order to compare the means, what distribution should we use? Earlier in this book we covered, at a glance, normal distribution and its characteristics, when we discussed how to check for normality previously in the book. Normal distribution returns a z-score. However, in practice, we would never use normal distribution. It is better to use t-distribution which approximates normal well.

The variance of the general population (of the world) is always unspecified and what we know is the variance of the samples; hence, we use t-distribution for comparing the means, which returns a t-score.

8.6 Degrees of Freedom

The larger the sample, the more similar the t-distribution to the normal distribution. We often encounter the term *degree of freedom* (df) in biostatistics. I believe the best way to explain and to digest it is from a mathematical point of view: if our sample is n, then the df is $n - 1$. Therefore, if we have a sample of $n = 10$ individuals, then df=9. Subtracting one unit from the sample accounts for the margin of error of the sample, which would always be different from the general population (N). The df resembles the size of the sample. The larger the sample, the higher the df.

Figure 8.2 below is obtained with the following code:

```
> x <- seq(-6, 6, length = 100)
> df = c(2,5,10,30)
> colour = c("red", "orange", "blue", "yellow","black")
> plot(x, dnorm(x), type = "l", lty = 2, xlab = "t-value", ylab =
"Density", main = "Comparison of t-distributions", col = "black")
> for (i in 1:4){ lines(x, dt(x, df[i]), col = colour[i])}
> legend("topright", c("d.f. = 2", "d.f. = 5", "d.f. = 10", "d.f.
= 30", "Normal"),
        col = colour, title = "t-distributions", lty = c(1,1,1,1,2))
```

Let us skip, for the moment, the explanation of the lengthy code and focus on the plot:

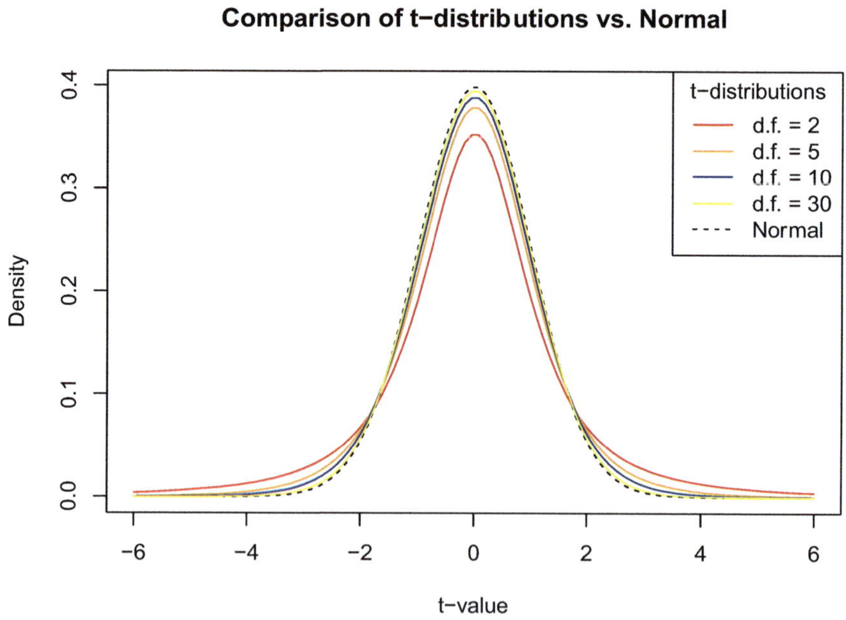

Fig. 8.2 Normal distribution and t-distributions with different degrees of freedom. As the sample size increases, t-distribution approaches normal distribution

I plot four curves that represent t-distribution with df of 2, 5, 10 and 30. The dotted curve represents the normal distribution. It is noteworthy that as the df gets bigger, because the sample size increases, the more the t-distribution resembles the normal distribution.

Again, we may always use the t-distribution for comparing the mean. This is specific for both small and large sample sizes.

8.7 Critical Value

We now discuss the *critical value*, for both the normal distribution and the t-distribution.

A *critical value* is a number or a point on a test distribution that we compare to the test statistic to determine whether or not to reject the null hypothesis. If the value of our test statistic is more extreme than the critical value, we can reject the null hypothesis and declare statistical significance.

This concept will become clearer later in this chapter.

For the time being we can say here that the critical value depends on:

i.) Level of significance (the alpha)
ii.) One or two-tailed test
iii.) Test distribution in use (i.e. *z*, *t* or *chi-squared* distribution)

As we said, the critical value of a distribution simply divides the distribution itself in an area of rejection (the upper and/or lower tail) and an area called *fail to reject*.

Let us assume that we know the standard deviation σ of the general population (*N*), and we know that individuals from the general population bleed 700 mL with a standard deviation of 150 mL after surgery.

According to our example data, in our sample (*n*) people in the Broccoli group bleed 475.3 mL. How extreme is my sample population test? Is my sample parameter statistically different from the general population?

Since we assume we know the variance of the general population, we can use a z-distribution and calculate the z-score:

$$z = \frac{\overline{x} - \mu}{\sigma} = \frac{475.3 - 700}{150} = -1.49$$

Whereas μ is the population mean, $\overline{x}$ is the sample mean and σ is the population known as the standard deviation. Our z-score is -1.49. The z-score says that our sample is -1.49 below the mean.

We should now locate this number in the normal z-distribution. In medicine the alpha level is almost often set as 0.05 (again, the alpha or significance level helps to specify the size of the region where the null hypothesis should be rejected).

However, before locating our z-score in the normal distribution to identify whether to accept or reject the null hypothesis, we should make some reflections about our statistical hypothesis. Are we hypothesising that the population parameter is different? Or greater or lower than the population mean?

8.8 One- or Two-Tailed Test

When we read the statistical part of medical papers, often we come across *one-tail* or *two-tailed* test definitions in the statistical test (e.g. a two-tailed t-test). It is in fact important to focus on the *direction* and *number* of tails. There are three scenarios for hypothesis testing: *greater than*, *lower than* and *not equal*.

For a normal distribution, the critical value for an alpha level of 0.05/95% confidence interval is 1.96 (this is where the rejection area begins). This is always the same, and normal distribution does not say anything about degree of freedom (Fig. 8.3).

If we look at the normal distribution, we may notice that the critical value with alpha 0.05 is ±1.96 from the centre for a two-tailed test, where the probability of 0.05 is divided between the two tails (0.025 each). Two-tailed refers to the fact that we are interested whether the value can be greater or less than the general population. If our question is whether the parameter would be lower or greater, then it is a one-tailed test. As you probably already understand, pretty much all hypothesis testing in medicine is based on two-tailed philosophy.

1.96 is the critical value for alpha level 0.05/95% confidence interval and two-tailed test. There are tables (not shown in this book) that will tell us the critical value for a given alpha level for a one- or two-tailed test. However, since in medicine we always use a two-tailed test with alpha 0.05/95% confidence interval, 1.96 is the number (the critical value) that we must remember.

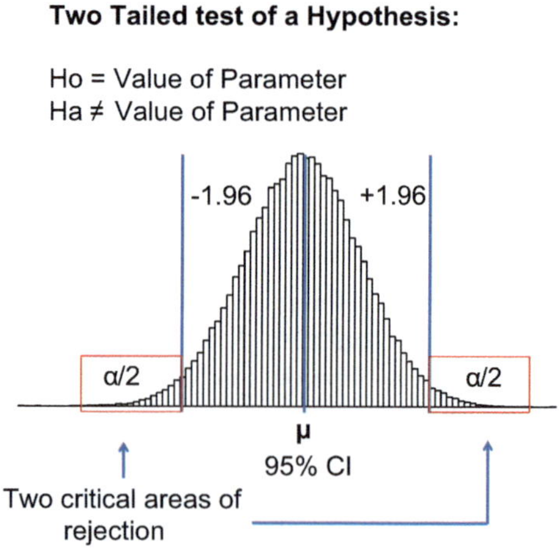

Fig. 8.3 Normal distribution with two-tailed rejection area. The alpha value is the significance level and helps to specify the size of the region where the null hypothesis should be rejected. For two-tailed, the alpha is divided by two (0.025 both sides)

Going back to our z-score test, we know it is −1.49. In the context of a two-tailed test hypothesis, this is less than the critical value of −1.96; hence, our t-test is located in the no-rejection area. We then fail to reject the null hypothesis (i.e. the bleeding is not statistically different from the general population).

8.9 t-Test, One and Two Tails

Z-distribution is unrealistic since we do not work with the general population, for which variance is unknown. We in fact work with *samples* from the general population. Thereby the t-distribution should always be used.

If we go back to our study on the effect of `Broccoli` on `Bleeding`, we calculated that the mean post-operative `Bleeding` of the n patients who included `Broccoli` in their diet before surgery was 475.3 mL, with 581 mL of `Bleeding` in the control (`noBroccoli`) group.

My null hypothesis is that the parameter `Bleeding` (μ) in the population is 581 mL, and I want to investigate if `Bleeding` differs in the two populations.

When I investigate the amount of post-operative `Bleeding` of my group of interest, there are only three possibilities for sets or pairs of hypothesis statements:

1. H_0: $\mu = 581$ mL
   H_a: $\mu \neq 581$ mL
   The amount of Bleeding in the Broccoli group (being 475.3 mL) is not equal to 581 mL; it could have been either less or greater than the control or population (two-tailed).
2. H_0: $\mu \leq 581$ mL
   H_a: $\mu > 581$ mL
   Means the amount of `Bleeding` in the `Broccoli` group is greater than the control (right tailed).
3. H_0: $\mu \geq 581$ mL
   H_a: $\mu < 581$ mL
   Means the amount of `Bleeding` in the `Broccoli` group is less than the control (left tailed).

Let us review the three hypothesis statements. The first option is the *two-tailed test*, and it is bidirectional by definition. When I started thinking about the effect of `Broccoli` on `Bleeding`, I hypothesised that the vegetables could have a protective effect on `Bleeding`, but I would not know a priori if `Broccoli` could have no effect at all (i.e. increase or decrease the amount of `Bleeding` in both directions).

By setting the hypothesis test as the first option ($H_0 : \mu = 581$ mL/$H_a : \mu \neq 581$ mL), we take into account the statistical possibility that `Bleeding` could either be higher or lower than the control population.

Similarly to the normal distribution, the two-tailed test distribution has two critical/rejection areas: right/positive side and left/negative side. It implies that our

`Bleeding` parameter may be greater or less than the control (the null hypothesis) or equal.

Note that the alternative hypothesis never contains *equality*; vice versa the null hypothesis always does. In fact, some use only an equal sign to denote the null.

Before calculating the t-test, to find out if the two means are different, let us review the crucial steps of hypothesis testing.

8.10 Crucial Steps

Researchers and statisticians use hypothesis testing to formally and mathematically check whether the hypothesis is true or false. To do so, the following steps must be carried out:

1. State the hypothesis: compose the research question (e.g. the earth is flat/ bisoprolol lowers systolic blood pressure).
2. Formulate a statistical analysis plan (SAP): devise how to collect samples, and decide the parameter and which distribution and test to use.
3. Analyse data: perform calculations described in the SAP.
4. Interpret the result.

The p-value is a number which indicates if our test is significant. In statistics, the p-value can be defined as the probability of obtaining results at least as extreme as the observed results of a statistical hypothesis test, assuming that the null hypothesis is correct. The level of significance is denoted by alpha. More specifically, alpha is the probability of rejecting the null when the null is true. A common mistake is to interpret the p-value as the probability that the null hypothesis is true.

Alpha and p-value are not the same:

Alpha: sets the standard for how extreme the data must be before we can reject the null hypothesis and is the probability of incorrectly rejecting a true null hypothesis. If we set the alpha level of a hypothesis test at 0.05, it means if we were to repeat the test many times, we would expect to incorrectly reject the null in about 5% of the tests.

p-Value: indicates *how extreme* the data is. p-Values tell the probability of obtaining an effect at least as large as the one we actually observed in the sample data.

In our example experiment, the p-value obtained with independent t-test was very low: <0.01. This is the probability of obtaining a sample mean (475.3 mL) that is at least as extreme as our sample mean in both tails of the distribution if the population mean is 581.7 mL.

With a 95% confidence interval, a small p-value (≤ 0.05) indicates strong evidence against the null; hence, we must reject the null and consider the alternative hypothesis as true. Note that a p-value greater than 0.05 would indicate weak evidence against the null; hence, we would fail to reject the null.

8.11 t-Test

We have three kinds of t-test:

i.) One sample t-test
ii.) Independent t-test
iii.) Paired t-test

One sample t-test compares the sample population mean to the mean (μ) of the general population with unknown standard deviation.

Independent t-test compares the mean of a sample population with another mean of an independent sample population with equal or unequal variance.

Paired t-test compares the mean of a group with the mean of the same group after a certain treatment.

We will discuss them all one by one.

8.12 Conducting One Sample t-Test in "R"

We have stated that there are three possible t-tests in statistics: one sample, paired and independent. The paired typically represents the differences between a pre- and post-test (i.e. quality of life measured before and after surgery in the same group) and independent is the comparison between two groups (e.g. mean post-operative `Bleeding` in the Broccoli vs noBroccoli group) where the variance can be different between the two groups. The two aforementioned t-tests (paired and independent) are the most used ones. However, there are situations where it is necessary to use the one sample t-test.

Remember that all of the three tests can be one- or two-tailed. It depends on our clinical question.

Let us go back to the `Broccoli` group and calculate the mean post-operative `Bleeding` along with the standard deviation:

```
> Broccoli<-MMstat[MMstat$Broccoli=='y',] # I created with basic
sub-setting the Broccoli group
> dim(Broccoli) # The group contains 203 individuals with 18
variables
[1] 203  18
> mean(broccoli$Bleeding)# Calculating the mean
[1] 475.3
> sd(broccoli$Bleeding)# and the standard deviation of my sample
Broccoli
[1] 114.8
```

Notably, I create the population Broccoli using the basic "R" function for subsetting `MMstat[MMstat$Broccoli=='y',]`. However, the same process could be achieved with the `filter( )` function in `dplyr` in the `tidyverse` R-package:

```
> mmsubset<-as_tibble(MMstat)
> Broccoli<-filter(mmsubset, Broccoli=='y')
```

We know that on average, individuals in the `Broccoli` group (n = 203) bled 475.3 mL ± 114.8 mL. Is this a large amount of bleeding? Let's compare to what is available in literature. We pretend to know that after cardiac surgery, on average individuals tend to bleed 670 mL of blood during the first 24 h. Now we would like to know if `Bleeding` in the `Broccoli` group (475.3 mL) is significantly lower than 670 mL. In order to do that, I need to run a one sample t-test and I would need the following information:

- **μ:** the mean of the comparison group, in this case what is available from literature about post-operative bleeding = 670 mL
- **$\bar{x}$:** the mean post-operative bleeding of our group of interest = 475.3 mL
- **s:** the standard deviation of bleeding in our Broccoli sample = 114.8 mL
- **n:** the number of observations in the Broccoli sample = 203

We now state our hypothesis: we would like to know if `Bleeding` in the `Broccoli` group is *less than* the one published in literature:

H_0: μ ≥ 670 mL (the null)

H_a: μ < 670 mL (the alternative)

Please note that the null and alternative hypotheses are mathematically opposite and we never use the ≥ in the alternative, always in the null. What we need to also specify is the level of significance (most commonly .05) and the degree of freedom (df). The latter can be difficult to explain, but as previously set out, from a mathematical point of view, it is very easy to define as n-1. Therefore, in this case the df = 203 − 1 = 202. Do also note the s refers to the standard deviation of bleeding in the sample (the `Broccoli` group) rather than the overall population. The standard deviation for the overall population is generally unknown. We now have all the elements to compute a one sample (left tail) t-test and we need to calculate the test statistic and find the critical value:

Calculate the test statistic (t):

$$t = \frac{\bar{x} - \mu}{\frac{s}{\sqrt{n}}} = \frac{475.3 - 670}{\frac{114.8}{\sqrt{203}}} = -24.14$$

Our test statistic is −24.14. We need to understand how this number compares to the critical value for $t_{\alpha=0.05,\ df=202}$, which means that we need to find the critical value with an alpha level of 0.05 and a degree of freedom (n − 1) of 202. Again, note that since we are running a one-tail (left) t-test, the entire alpha level (0.05) will be on one side.

8.13 How to Find *t* Critical Values

After we calculate the test statistic, to determine if the result is statistically significant, we need to compare it to a *t critical value*. If the value of the test statistic is greater than the *t critical value*, then the result of the test is statistically significant.

This process is identical to the one we conducted for the normal distribution. Except in this case the critical value depends also on the df, and if $df \to \infty$ then the t-distribution approaches normal.

How do we find the t critical value? Simply by using a t-distribution table or using "R". Set out below is an example of t-distribution. To determine the critical value for our scenario, alpha=0.05, df=202, one-tailed test, we need to find the number that is the interception between the corresponding *df* and *alpha level* (Fig. 8.4):

As an example from Fig. 8.4, for df = 1, alpha level = 0.05, one-tailed test, the critical value is 6.3. Obviously, the chart cannot show infinite degrees of freedom. We will use the `qt()` function in "R" to find the critical value that corresponds to our desired df:

```
> qt(p=.05, df=202, lower.tail=TRUE)
[1] -1.652432
```

The `qt` function requires the `p=` significant level, the `df=` of our sample and the type of `tail`.

We now know that the test statistic is −24.14 and the critical value is −1.65. For any value below −1.65 we should reject the null hypothesis (H_0: $\mu \geq 670$ mL) and state that the bleeding in the Broccoli group is significantly lower than 670 mL, since the t-statistic falls in the rejection area.

Let us scrutinise the curve below to better understand the relationship between the test statistic and the critical value (Fig. 8.5):

Note that to find the critical value for the right tail, we should use:

	P						
one-tail	0.1	0.05	0.025	0.01	0.005	0.001	0.0005
two-tails	0.2	0.1	0.05	0.02	0.01	0.002	0.001
DF							
1	3.078	6.314	12.706	31.821	63.656	318.289	636.578
2	1.886	2.92	4.303	6.965	9.925	22.328	31.6
3	1.638	2.353	3.182	4.541	5.841	10.214	12.924
4	1.533	2.132	2.776	3.747	4.604	7.173	8.61
5	1.476	2.015	2.571	3.365	4.032	5.894	6.869
6	1.44	1.943	2.447	3.143	3.707	5.208	5.959
7	1.415	1.895	2.365	2.998	3.499	4.785	5.408

Fig. 8.4 *t*-Distribution table

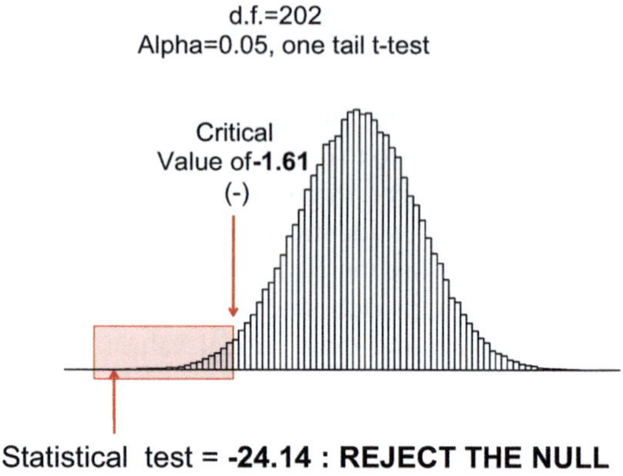

Fig. 8.5 *t*-Distribution with area of rejection; the t-score (−24.14) falls in the area of rejection since it is lower than the critical value of −1.61

```
> qt(p=.05, df=202, lower.tail=FALSE)
```

and for two tails we must divide the alpha by two, since we need to distribute the alpha level between the two tails:

```
> qt(p=.05/2, df=202, lower.tail=FALSE)
```

8.14 Using "R" Code for Conducting One Sample *t*-Test

Obviously, things are easier when using "R" and we can directly run the one sample t-test using the `t.test` function and specifying the `broccoli$Bleeding` vector and the mean of the population (`mu=670`) as follows:

```
> t.test(broccoli$Bleeding, mu=670, lower.tail=TRUE, conf.
level = 0.95)
```

```
    One Sample t-test
data:  broccoli$Bleeding
t = -24.14, df = 202, p-value < 0.01
alternative hypothesis: true mean is not equal to 670
95 percent confidence interval: 459.48 491.27
sample estimates: mean of x  475.37
```

The function returns everything we need to know, the t statistic, *p*-value and 95% confidence interval. Again, we can confirm that 459 mL is significantly lower than 670 m and reject the null hypothesis.

8.15 Independent t-Test

Independent t-test is used when we need to compare the mean of two different groups. Using our example experiment to demonstrate, say we would like to compare the means of the post-operative bleeding from the Broccoli and noBroccoli groups. The groups must be mutually exclusive. Also, independent t-test is a parametric test; hence, the assumption of normality is required. However, according to the central limit theory, when working with a sample that is large enough, we may use a parametric test independently from the nature of the sample.

From a statistical point of view, since we are dealing with two samples, the formula for the independent t-test differs from that of the one sample test and also the computation of the df:

$$t = \frac{\left(\overline{x}_1 - \overline{x}_2\right)}{S_p\sqrt{\frac{1}{n_1} + \frac{1}{n_2}}}$$

The numerator, as expected, is the difference between the two groups' averages. The denominator is an estimate of the standard error of the difference between the two unknown population means.

S_p is the *pooled standard deviation*. This is specific, since we have two samples. It is calculated as per the formula below:

$$s_p^2 = \frac{\left((n_1 - 1)s_1^2\right) + \left((n_2 - 1)s_2^2\right)}{n_1 + n_2 - 2}$$

And the df:

$$df = n_1 + n_2 - 2$$

You do not need to remember the formulas by heart because "R" calculates it for you. However, it is important to check if the variance between the two samples differs.

To check the homogeneity of the variance, we will use the `bartlett.test` and `list( )` functions:

```
> bartlett.test(list(broccoli$Bleeding, nobroccoli$Bleeding))

    Bartlett test of homogeneity of variances
data:  list(broccoli$Bleeding, nobroccoli$Bleeding)
Bartlett's K-squared = 56.22, df = 1, p-value = <0.01
```

By comparing the variance, the test returns a significant p-value; hence, we should reject the null hypothesis (variance is homogeneous).

We can now run the `t.test` specifying the variance as not equal, as set out below:

```
> t.test(broccoli$Bleeding, nobroccoli$Bleeding, paired = FALSE,
alternative = 'two.sided', var.equal = FALSE)

Welch Two Sample t-test

data: broccoli$Bleeding and nobroccoli$Bleeding
t = -7.75, df = 490.71, p-value = <0.01
alternative hypothesis: true difference in means is not equal to 0
95 percent confidence interval: -133.25 -79.38
sample estimates: mean of x mean of y 475.37 581.70
```

By setting the variance as not equal, "R" returns Welch's test rather than the conventional t-test. Welch's test is also named unequal variance t-test and is practically an adaptation of the t-test. It is more reliable when the two samples have different variance or unequal sample size. While Welch's t-test is designed for unequal variance, the assumption of normality should still hold.

8.16 Troubleshooting with Independent t-Test

Very often in medicine we deal with non-normal distribution. One of the factors that may determine non-normality in a sample is the presence of the outliers. In fact, in our sample we do have some of them that may render the analysis slightly more complicated. If we boxplot the observation we will notice many outliers. In this case, even with the sample being large enough, and according to the central limit theory, we may use a parametric t-test. However, a non-parametric test would definitely fit better instead. Let us plot and visualise the distribution of the *bleeding* observation with (Fig. 8.6):

```
> ggplot(MMstat, aes(x=Broccoli, y=Age, color-Broccoli)) +theme_
bw()+ geom_boxplot() + geom_jitter(shape = 16,
position=position_jitter(0.3))
```

The boxplot analysis is definitely showing many outliers. In this case we may accept violation of normality and proceed with non-parametric tests. In this case we can use the Wilcoxon test.

There are two types of Wilcoxon test:

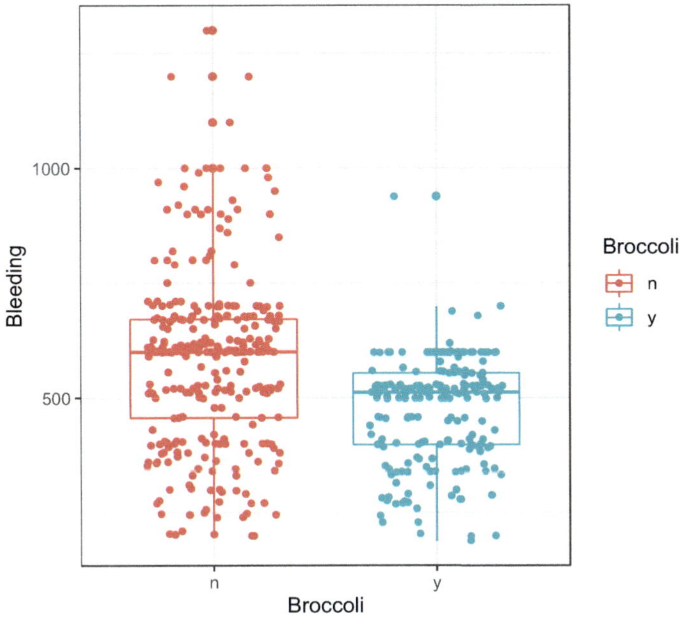

Fig. 8.6 Post-operative bleeding grouped by the variable "Broccoli" with evidence of non-normal distribution

1. The Mann-Whitney-Wilcoxon test (also known as the Wilcoxon rank sum test) which is performed when the samples are independent (essentially this test is the non-parametric equivalent to the Student's t-test for *independent* samples).
2. The Wilcoxon signed-rank test (also sometimes referred to as the Wilcoxon test for paired samples; see paragraph below) which is performed when the samples are paired/dependent (the non-parametric equivalent to the Student's t-test for *paired* samples).

The `wilcox.test( )` function for both is the same, but the coding is different; we must specify if the sample is paired or not.

8.17 Paired or Dependent t-Test

Dependent t-test is a parametric test that compares the mean of the same group at two different time points. Our fictitious example experiment means the dataset `MMstat` does not contain such variables measured at two different time points. A common example is when you administer a test at baseline (e.g. a test that measures the quality of life) and then you repeat the same test at a certain point after surgery. The other two t-test (one sample and two sample independent) tails can be one (greater than *or* less than) or two-sided (greater than *and* less than).

Let us create two vectors: sBP1 which contains measurements of systolic blood pressure of ten individuals before treatment and sBP2 which contains the same measurements after 1 month of therapy with bisoprolol, a beta-blocker that has an effect on heart rate and blood pressure:

```
> sBP1<-c(140, 138, 129, 135, 145, 173, 183, 130, 101, 101) #sys-
tolic blood pressure mmHg at baseline
> sBP2<-c(120, 133, 123, 125, 125, 133, 123, 120, 99, 100) # sys-
tolic blood pressure measured in the same individuals 1 month after
therapy with Bisoprolol
```

If we run a boxplot analysis, we observe that the blood pressure is lower at the 1-month follow-up (Fig. 8.7):

```
> boxplot(sBP1, sBP2, col='yellow', main='systolic blood pressure')
```

We may now want to run the paired t-test to understand if there is any significant difference between the two groups:

H_0: $\mu = 0$ and the H_a: $\mu \neq 0$

As always, null and alternative are mathematically opposite.

```
> t.test(sBP1, sBP2, paired=TRUE, alternative ='two.sided')


     Paired t-test
data:  sBP1 and sBP2
t = 2.9007, df = 9, p-value = 0.01757
alternative hypothesis: true difference in means is not equal to 0
95 percent confidence interval: 3.830409 30.969591
sample estimates: mean of the differences 17.4
```

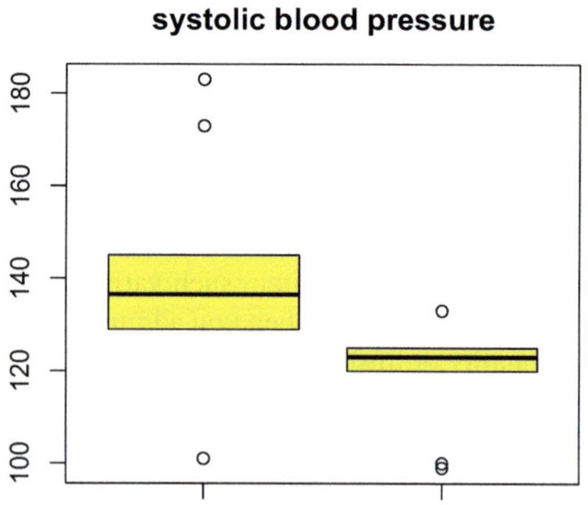

Fig. 8.7 Paired t-test boxplot showing blood pressure at baseline (left) and at 1 month

The paired t-test, as all the other t-tests, returns a t-value of 2.9 with a degree of freedom n − 1=9. As we learnt before, we can obtain a critical value from a t-distribution being alpha level 0.05/2 (two sided) and df = 9 with the below function:

```
> qt(p=.05/2, df=9, lower.tail=FALSE)
[1] 2.262157
```

The critical value is 2.26. We know that the critical value divides the rejection area from the non-rejection area. Our t-value is 2.9, higher (right side) than the critical value; thereby we should reject the null hypothesis. The p-value is automatically calculated by "R" and is p = 0.01. A trick to remember when to reject and not reject the null is: when the p-value is low the null must go; when the p-value is high the null must fly.

And for non-normally distributed values, we should use the Wilcoxon signed-rank test:

```
> wilcox.test(broccoli$Bleeding, nobroccoli$Bleeding, paired=TRUE,
alternative='two.sided', conf.int = 0.95)# we use wilcox.test for
not normally distributed data, paired=TRUE specifies that it is a
dependent t.test
```

8.18 t-Test in "R"

One-sample t-test:	one or two tails	
Compare the sample mean with the population mean. It can be one or two tails.		
`> t.test(broccoli$Bleeding, mu = 670, lower.tail=TRUE, conf.level = 0.95)# example of one tail one sample t.test. Comparing the mean of the bleeding of my sample Broccoli with a general population mean of 670 mL.`		
Two-sample t-test:	one or two tails	dependent or independent
– Independent t-test		
Independent t-test is used when we need to compare the means of two different groups. It can be one or two tails.		
Same size and/or same variance:		t.test
Different variance:		Welch test

```
> bartlett.test(list(broccoli$Bleeding,
nobroccoli$Bleeding))#use bartlett test for checking variance,
if variance not equal specify it in the t.test function and will
return the welch test.
> t.test(broccoli$Bleeding, nobroccoli$Bleeding, paired = FALSE,
alternative = 'two.sided', var.equal = FALSE)# we use
alternative = 'two.sided' or 'lower' or 'greater' to specify one
tail or two tails test
```

Non-normal distribution:	Mann-Whitney-Wilcoxon test

```
wilcox.test(broccoli$Bleeding, nobroccoli$Bleeding,
paired=FALSE, alternative='two.sided', conf.int = 0.95)# we us
wilcox.test for not normally distributed data, paired=FALSE
specify that is independent t.test
```

– Dependent t-test

Dependent t-test is used when we need to compare the means from the same group (e.g. two sets of measurements from the same population group pre- and post-treatment).

```
> t.test(sBP1, sBP2,paired=TRUE, alternative ='two.sided')#sBP1
and sBP2 represent blood pressure from the same group before and
after a treatment
```

Non-normal distribution:	Wilcoxon signed-rank test

```
wilcox.test(broccoli$Bleeding, nobroccoli$Bleeding, paired=TRUE,
alternative='two.sided', conf.int = 0.95)# we us wilcox.test
for not normally distributed data, paired=TRUE specify that is
dependent t.test
```

8.19 More on Non-parametric Tests

I want to discuss non-parametric tests in this chapter because, in medicine, we often encounter samples with non-normal distribution. Non-parametric tests (e.g. the `wilcox.test`) have the same objectives as their parametric counterparts. However, they have two main advantages over parametric tests: they do not require the assumption of normality of distributions, and, very importantly, they can deal with outliers.

You might wonder: *why don't we always use a non-parametric test, so we don't have to be preoccupied about testing for normality?*

The reason is that non-parametric tests (i.e. the `t.test`) are usually less powerful than the corresponding parametric tests when the normality assumption holds.

Importantly, with a non-parametric test (i.e. the `wilcox.test`) we are less likely to reject the null hypothesis when it is false if the data follows a normal distribution (type II error).

8.20 Chi-Squared Test of Independence and Fisher's Exact Test

We have discussed z-test and t-test and how both of them are used for numeric variables (the mean). In medicine we always use the t-test or the correspondent non-parametric version to compare the mean.

What about not numeric/categorical variables?

The chi-squared test of independence is a method for testing independence between two categorical variables.

Say we are interested in understanding whether or not there are more male individuals in the Broccoli vs noBroccoli group. Perhaps to find out if female or male patients are more prone to developing complications such as bleeding or in-hospital mortality. In order to perform the chi-squared test we should compute a contingency table (named 4 x 4 table), using the `table` function:

```
> table(MMstat$Male, MMstat$Broccoli)
      n   y
  0 158 118
  1 139  85
```

The function returns the distribution of gender by group (Broccoli/noBroccoli). For the `Broccoli` group (==y), we have 85 male (==1) and 118 female (==0).

Let's save the table within an object we call `chisex`:

```
> chisex<-table(MMstat$Male, MMstat$Broccoli)
```

And produce a barplot with the `barplot` function and the following code (Fig. 8.8):

```
> barplot(chisex, beside=T, legend=c("Female", "Male"),
col=c('green', 'yellow'), main='Sex distribution in the Broccoli
vs noBroccoli')
```

Visually, the barplot shows that in the *n* group (*n*=noBroccoli) there are more female than male. Similarly, in the *y* group (*y*=Broccoli) female are more represented.

Again, the question remains: is the proportion similar between the groups? We should now run a statistical test, such as the chi-squared test, using the `chisq.test` function:

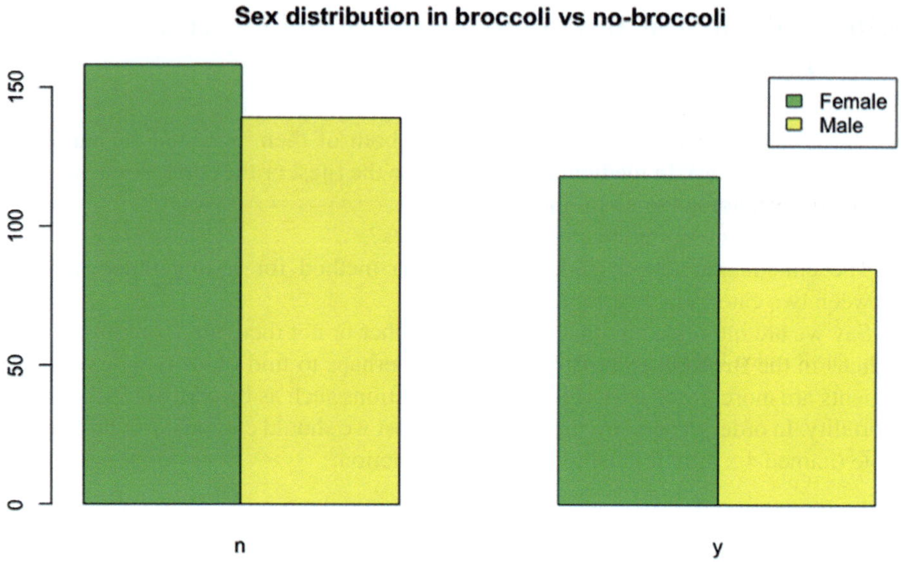

Fig. 8.8 Barplot visualisation of male and female proportions grouped by the Broccoli variable

```
> chisq.test(chisex)

    Pearson's Chi-squared test with Yates'
    continuity correction
data:   chisex X-squared = 0.99389, df = 1, p-value = 0.3188
```

The test returns an X-squared statistic and a p-value. In this case we fail to reject the null hypothesis. The distribution of gender between the Broccoli and noBroccoli groups does not statistically differ. The p-value is well above the alpha level of 0.05.

If the chi-squared assumptions are not met, we should then use the Fisher's exact test. The chi-squared test applies an approximation assuming that the sample size is large, while the Fisher's exact test runs an exact procedure for small sample size.

```
> fisher.test(chisex)

    Fisher's Exact Test for Count Data

data:   chisex p-value = 0.3139
alternative hypothesis: true odds ratio is not equal to 1 95 per-
cent confidence interval: 0.5616834 1.1923219
sample estimates: odds ratio 0.8191337
```

The Fisher's test confirms no difference of distribution between the groups returning also the odds ratio. We discuss in dedicated chapter later in the book what odds ratio and hazard ratio are.

8.21 Creating Matrices

Sometimes we only have proportions (raw numbers) and we want to build a contingency, 4 × 4 table. For example, let us assume we already know the number of individuals in the Broccoli ($n = 297$) and noBroccoli groups ($n = 203$) and the proportion of female gender such as 158 females in noBroccoli and 118 in Broccoli. That leaves us with 139 and 85 male in the noBroccoli and Broccoli groups, respectively. We would like to discover whether or not there are any significant differences.

To do so I need to build a matrix with the `matrix` function:

```
> chisexmat= matrix(c(158,118,139,85), nrow=2, ncol=2,
dimnames=list(c('Female', 'Male'), c('noBroccoli', 'Broccoli')))
```

We create a vector named `chisexmat` that is composed of four elements, number of females or males in each of the Broccoli and noBroccoli groups. The matrix is arranged with two rows `nrow=2` and two columns `ncol=2` and then names the rows and columns assigned with `dimnames`.

We can now perform a `chisq.test`:

```
> chisq.test(chisexmat)
    Pearson's Chi-squared test with Yates' continuity
    correction

data:  chisexmat
X-squared = 0.99389, df = 1, p-value = 0.3188
```

which returns X-squared statistic and p-value well above the alpha level. Hence, we fail to reject the null hypothesis.

8.22 Type I and Type II Error

In hypothesis testing we have two options:

1. *Reject the null hypothesis* (H_0) and conclude that there is sufficient evidence to overturn the established belief about the population parameter (e.g. we provide solid evidence against the earth being round).
2. *Fail to reject the null hypothesis* (H_0) and conclude that there is insufficient evidence to overturn the established value of the population parameter (e.g. we can't provide solid evidence supporting the earth being flat).

Is there any possibility that, when we conduct a study to demonstrate that the earth is flat, we can be wrong? When we conduct a study, we specify our alpha level

(level of significance), but the alpha level is also the probability of committing a type I error, also known as a *false positive*.

The important concept is that, in statistics, we always want to avoid a type I error, i.e. we should minimise the possibility to affirm that the earth is flat, while it is not. Before rejecting the *status quo* we should have really strong evidence against it. At the end of the day everything works and functions correctly on a rounded earth.

A similar analogy would be in court. Individuals are innocent until proven guilty, and theoretically it would be more detrimental to jail innocent people than to not jail truly guilty individuals. That is why the alpha level is strict. Type II error, intuitively, is to let the guilty person go. In that case the null hypothesis is false, but there is a failure to reject it.

	Null hypothesis is TRUE	Null hypothesis is FALSE
REJECT the null hypothesis	Type I error (false positive) - Alpha-	Correct outcome (true positive)
FAIL to reject the null hypothesis	Correct outcome (true negative)	Type II error (false negative) - Beta-

When we reject the TRUE NULL, we commit a type I error (i.e. we accept that the earth is flat, while it is not, or we jail an innocent individual).

When we fail to reject a FALSE NULL, we commit a type II error (we still keep the belief that the earth is rounded, while it is not, or we set a guilty individual free).

We should remember now that the probabilities of committing a type I error are alpha, and the probability of committing a type II error is beta, and 1-beta is known as the power of test. Type I error is very serious, more serious than type II. In fact, researchers always fix the probability of committing a type I error at 0.05 and sometimes at 0.01.

8.23 Conclusions

Hypothesis testing is a method of statistical inference. There are two opposite *worlds*: the *status quo* (H_0, the null hypothesis) and the *alternative to the status quo* (H_a, the alternative hypothesis) which is the research question that we want to validate. However, the null hypothesis is true and remains so unless very solid evidence is brought against it.

If the evidence against the null is valid, we then *reject the null*. If evidence is not valid, we *fail to reject the null*.

In statistics, the null is very well protected. We can't risk to reject the null (to accept the alternative) and to change the status quo unless we are extremely positively in favour of the alternative. That is why we generally set the so-called alpha level at 0.05.

The alpha level is the probability to reject the null when the null is true. This is also called a type I error. The alpha level 0.05 comes with a confidence interval of 1-alpha (95%). Setting the alpha at 0.05 with 95% confidence interval means we have 5% possibility of a type I error.

We conduct hypothesis testing to compare parameters of populations. Hypothesis tests are based on probability distributions. If we want to compare means, we can use the z-distribution (normal distribution) but more realistically the t-distribution.

Normal distribution is used when the standard deviation of the general population is known. t-Distribution is used when the standard deviation of the population is unknown and replaced by the standard deviation of the sample population. As the t-distribution increases in sample size, it approximates the normal distribution.

The t-test returns a t-statistic; the t-score is then compared to a critical value. The critical value delineates the rejection area (one or two tails) from the non-rejection area (the centre between the tails). The critical value depends on the number of tails (one or two tails) and on the degree of freedom. Finally, a p-value is obtained.

The p-value can be defined as the probability of obtaining results at least as extreme as the observed results of a statistical hypothesis test, assuming that the null hypothesis is correct.

There are three kinds of t-tests: one sample, independent and paired t-test. t-Tests are used to compare means. They can be one- or two-tailed, depending on the direction chosen (greater/right, less/left, not equal, both sided). t-Tests require a normality assumption. Also, equal variance is expected; if not the Welch test is preferred. If samples are non-normally distributed, we may consider to use the Mann-Whitney-Wilcoxon test. Finally, the chi-squared test is used to compare categorical variables.

Further Readings

Biau DJ, Jolles BM, Porcher R. P value and the theory of hypothesis testing: an explanation for new researchers. Clin Orthop Relat Res. 2010;468(3):885–92. https://doi.org/10.1007/s11999-009-1164-4.

Guyatt G, Jaeschke R, Httteddle N, Cook D, Shannon H, Walter S. Basic statistics for clinicians: 1. Hypothesis testing. CMAJ. 1995;152(1):27–32.

Hazra A, Gogtay N. Biostatistics series module 2: overview of hypothesis testing. Indian J Dermatol. 2016;61(2):137–45. https://doi.org/10.4103/0019-5154.177775.

Kim HY. Statistical notes for clinical researchers: Chi-squared test and Fisher's exact test. Restor Dent Endod. 2017;42(2):152–5. https://doi.org/10.5395/rde.2017.42.2.152. Epub 2017 Mar 30

Tenny S, Abdelgawad I. Statistical significance. 2021 Nov 23. In: StatPearls [Internet]. Treasure Island, FL: StatPearls Publishing; 2022.

Vyas D, Balakrishnan A, Vyas A. The value of the <i>P</i> value. Am J Robot Surg. 2015;2(1):53–6. https://doi.org/10.1166/ajrs.2015.1017.

Chapter 9
Linear Regression

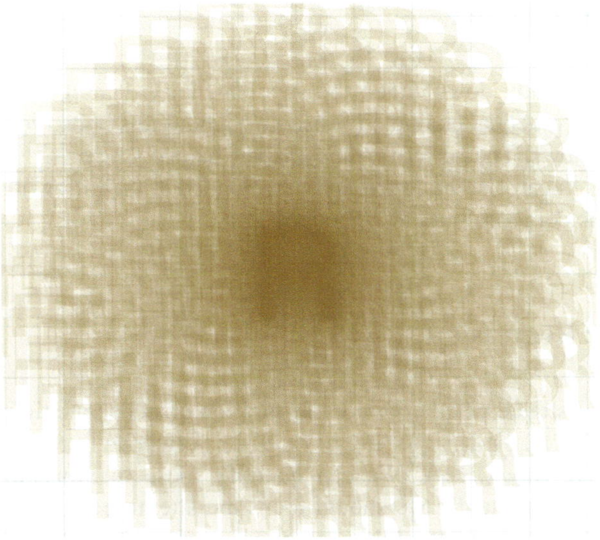

9.1 Software and R-Packages Required for This Chapter

If you haven't already, you need to download and install base-R and R-studio as set out in Chap. 2 under the heading "Downloading "R" and R-studio".

M. Moscarelli, *Biostatistics With 'R': A Guide for Medical Doctors*,
https://doi.org/10.1007/978-3-031-33073-5_9

The relevant R-packages needed for this chapter are:

- tidyverse—it can be downloaded at:
  http://tidyverse.tidyverse.org
- sjPlot—it can be downloaded at:
  https://strengejacke.github.io/sjPlot
- rms—it can be downloaded at:
  https://github.com/harrelfe/rms
- gridExtra—it can be downloaded at:
  Repository: CRAN
- MASS—it can be downloaded at:
  http://www.stats.ox.ac.uk/pub/MASS4

9.2 Where to Download the Example Dataset and Script for This Chapter

If you haven't already downloaded the supplementary dataset named `MMstat.csv` created as a practical example for use throughout this book, you will find it at the link that follows. The script for this chapter named `Chapter 9. Linear regression.R` can also be found and downloaded at the following link:

https://github.com/mmlondon77/Biobook.git.

9.3 Linear Regression

How can we investigate whether or not the duration of ischaemic time `CC` increases the post-operative `Bleeding` or if `Broccoli` is effective in reducing the length of post-operative stay (`LOS`)? We can quantify these relationships with linear regression. Most importantly we should focus the attention on the fact that linear regression is an analysis method that can be used when the outcome of interest is continuous. In this case, linear regression analysis is appropriate since our outcome of interest is numeric and continuous (i.e. amount of bleeding, days of post-operative stay).

This is different from logistic regression, where the outcome of interest is binary (i.e. dead/alive after surgery, re-explored or not re-explored after surgery, etc.).

In Chap. 7 about correlation, I specified that correlation (i.e. Pearson's correlation) is a measure of strength. You may remember that Pearson's correlation r is a kind of statistical guide, and anything greater than 0.7 is interpreted as strong, 0.5 as moderate and 0.3 as weak. However, with linear regression we are interested in the description and quantification of the relationship (i.e. duration of the ischaemic time and amount of post-operative bleeding), and more specifically the aim is to use one variable (e.g. `Broccoli`) to predict the other (e.g. `Bleeding`).

What is a *dependent variable*? The dependent variable (also referred to as the outcome of interest or response variable) is in fact what we are interested in and what we want to measure (the outcome *y*). The *independent variable* (also called explanatory variable or predictor *x*) is that which may influence the dependent variable *y*.

The dependent variable is represented on the y-axis while the explanatory variable on the x-axis. This is not very important for correlation, but is in fact mandatory for linear regression analysis.

In simple linear regression we include one explanatory variable (*x*), while in multiple linear regression we include many explanatory variables (*x*).

This concept (simple/multiple regression—dependent and independent variables) is similar to logistic regression and to Cox regression for survival analysis.

9.4 How Linear Regression Works

To better explain how linear regression works, I revert back to correlation.

We have already seen the plot in the correlation chapter and how it was obtained with the code (Fig. 9.1):

```
>    plot(MMstat$Bleeding~MMstat$CC,    col=c('blue',    'green'), xlab='Cross clamp or ischemic time min', ylab='Bleeding ml')
```

```
> abline(lm(MMstat$Bleeding~MMstat$CC), col="red")
```

The regression line shown in the right plot above in red (obtained using the `abline( )` command) is the straight line that minimises the distances of all the observations from the straight line itself (optimal straight line). It quantifies the

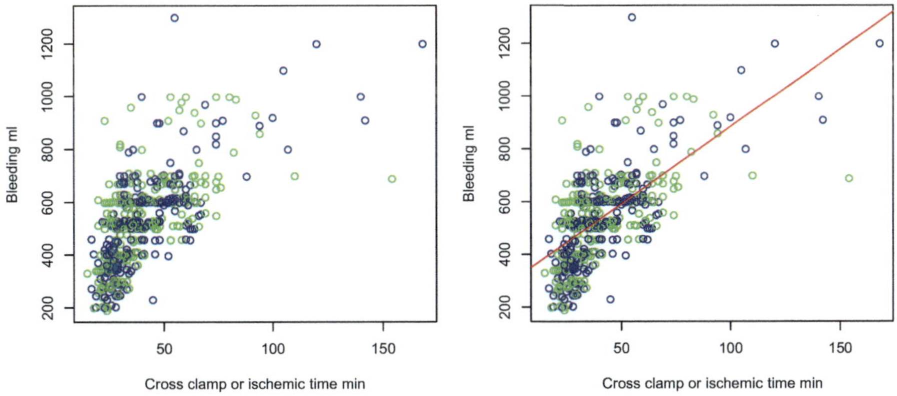

Fig. 9.1 Correlation between cross-clamp and post-operative bleeding (the red line is the line of best fit)

relationship between the two variables, in this scenario `CC` on the x-axis and `Bleeding` on the y-axis.

The distance between each observation and the straight red line is called *residual*.

The plot in Fig. 9.2 shows a few residuals (black lines that connect the observation to the line of best fit) on the upper right side of the figure (the plot in Fig. 9.2 is produced with base-R):

Residuals are calculated by subtracting the *fitted value* (also known as *predicted value*) from the *observed value*:

$$e_i\,(\text{residual}) = y_i\,(\text{observed value}) - \hat{y}_i\,(\text{fitted value})$$

The fitted value corresponds to the red line that is the best fit. The observed value is in fact what we observe in reality in analysis.

As in the previous chapter, I use both basic graph and `ggplot2` to visualise residuals.

Let us use `ggplot2` to visualise all the residuals vs fitted (Fig. 9.3):

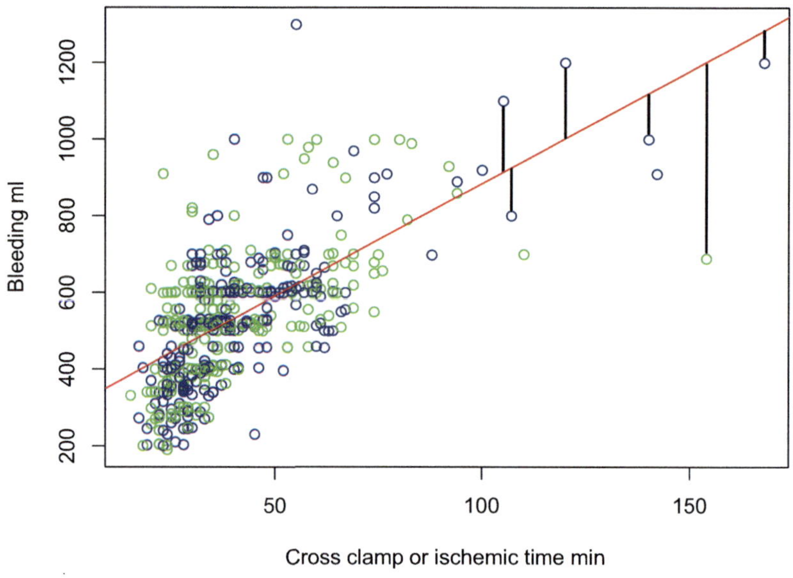

Fig. 9.2 Residuals are the distances from the observed and fitted values

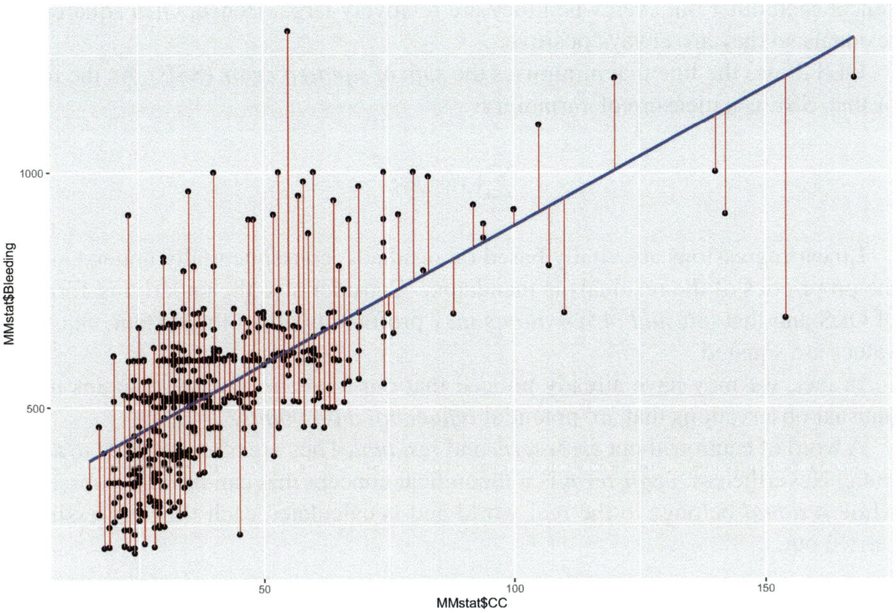

Fig. 9.3 Residuals shown with library broom and ggplot2

```
> library(broom)# we are using the library broom that belongs to
tidyverse
> model.diag.metrics <- augment(model)
> ggplot(model.diag.metrics , aes(MMstat$CC, MMstat$Bleeding)) +
  geom_point() +
  stat_smooth(method = lm, se = FALSE) +
 geom_segment(aes(xend = MMstat$CC, yend = .fitted), color = "red",
size = 0.3)
```

It goes without saying that Fig. 9.3 better depicts the residuals than the previous Fig. 9.2. Note in Fig. 9.3 the line of best fit is in blue.

How do we calculate the line of best fit? There are various ways, but the standard approach is the method called *least squares regression (OLS: ordinary least squared).*

The least square method fits a regression line that minimises the sum of the squared vertical distances between the observed value and the fitted line. Why squared? Since some residuals will be negative, they must be squared for calculation. We can't merely sum the residuals, since positive and negative values will cancel each other out even when they are relatively large. Hence, OLS squares the residuals so they are always positive.

OLS draws the line that minimises the *sum of squared error* (SSE). As the result of that, SSE is a measure of variability:

$$\sum_{i=1}^{n}(y_i - \hat{y}_i)^2$$

Linear regressions are vitally based on residuals; consequentially understanding the proprieties of the residuals is mandatory. Consider also the underlying formula of OLS and that *unusual observations* may profoundly affect the system, since the values are squared.

In fact, we may have already noticed that our `MMstat` dataset contains many unusual observations that are potential *influential data points*.

A word of caution about *error term* and *residual*. They are often referred to as the same. Nevertheless, *error term* is a theoretical concept that can never be observed, while *residual* belongs to the real world and is calculated each time regression is carried out.

9.5 Linear Regression Formula and Simple Linear Regression

Below is the simplified formula for one single predictor:

$$y = \alpha + \beta x + \varepsilon$$

- ***y*** is the dependent variable.
- ***α*** is where the regression line crosses the y-axis (the intercept).
- ***β*** is the slope (when $x = 0$, you can see from the equation that y will simply equal alpha, and the beta term will disappear).
- ***x*** is the independent/explanatory variable.
- **ε** is the error terms.

Let us assume that we would like to quantify the relationship between the dependent `Bleeding` variable and the independent `CC` (cross-clamp/ischaemic time) variable. Those in fact are the ones already plotted in Figs. 9.2 and 9.3: `Bleeding` on the y-axis (dependent variable) and `CC` on the x-axis (independent variable). Since the outcome of interest (`Bleeding`) is continuous, we can compute linear regression using the `lm( )` function:

```
> mymodel<-lm(MMstat$Bleeding~MMstat$CC)# lm stands for lin-
ear model
> summary(mymodel)
Coefficients:
             Estimate Std. Error t value Pr(>|t|)
(Intercept) 297.87     14.20     20.96   <0.01
MMstat$CC     5.87      0.31     18.63   <0.01

> confint(mymodel)
                2.5 %    97.5 %
(Intercept) 269.96 325.79
MMstat$CC     5.25   6.49
```

The `summary` function returns the following helpful information about the model constructed:

- The `Estimate` (the regression coefficient, which includes β and α) which represents the slope of the regression line
- The `Standard error`, which shows how much variation there is around the estimates of the regression coefficient
- The `t value` (test statistic) which is the t-value from a two-sided t-test (whereby the larger the test statistic, the less likely it is the results occurred by chance)
- The `p-value (Pr(>|t|))` which shows how likely the calculated t-value would have occurred by chance if the null hypothesis of no effect were true

Then the `confint` function returns the 95% confidence interval.

As a reminder, the ~ symbol is an operator which sets out the relationship between the independent variable and the dependent variable. This operator is crucial for regression.

Beta tells us how much, on average, the outcome variable increases in mL for every 1 unit increase in the x variable.

In our simple model, beta is 5.8 (the β coefficient), which means that with every 1-minute increase in cross-clamp, we predict the average bleeding will increase by 5.8 mL. We could also say that with every 10-minute increase, the bleeding increases by 58 mL. The increases are given in the unit of measures of both the variables *mL/minute*, *mL* for the dependent `Bleeding` variable and *minute* for the independent `CC` variable.

α is the bleeding value we would expect for individuals who have *zero* cross-clamp time. This is an example of where α does not provide a meaningful estimate (i.e. we cannot have zero cross-clamp time in cardiac surgery unless other approaches are considered, and in this case our example dataset does not contain any observations from surgeries without cross-clamp). Importantly, we should never use this model to predict *outside the range of observed data.*

The `confint` function returns the 95% confident interval (CI). The wider the CI, the more uncertain we are about the true population parameter. In our case the β coefficient is 5.87 with a relatively small 95% CI: 5.25–6.49. Importantly, the 95%

CI does not include 0; it means that the result is significant, with a significance level of 0.05 and with a p-value of <0.01.

In this first example of simple linear regression, I arbitrarily selected a continuous variable as the independent/explanatory variable (the `CC`/cross-clamp or ischaemic time). This was for the sake of simplicity since it is more informative plotting two numerical variables together.

However, the main research question is whether the `Broccoli` variable influences post-operative `Bleeding`. Luckily, a linear model can also accommodate the dichotomous `Broccoli=='y'` and `Broccoli=='n'` variable, as you will see over the next few paragraphs.

9.6 More About the Intercept

I specified that α is the intercept (also called the constant) where the regression line crosses/intercepts the y-axis. From a mathematical point of view, it is also defined as the *mean dependent value* when all the other independent variables equal zero. Nevertheless, a scenario where all the explanatory variables would be zero is hardly ever observed. Very often the constant is meaningless, yet must be included in regression analysis. You should also keep in mind that often the intercept can be located outside the observed values.

I reiterate as a general statistical guideline we should never make predictions outside the observed data. However, the intercept should always be included in the regression model.

9.7 Model Assumption

So far, the initial model we have built `mymodel<-lm(MMstat$Bleeding~MMstat$CC)` is very simple. Later we add more variables to see an example of a more advanced model (multivariable regression).

Please note that often people misuse the term *multivariate regression. Multivariate* refers to a scenario where we should evaluate multiple outcomes at once (this is very rarely the case), whereas *multivariable* refers to many predictors included in a model.

For the moment we focus on this simplified model made from only one predictor (`CC`).

There are three assumptions we make when fitting a linear regression model:

1. The relationship between the independent and the dependent variable is approximately linear.
2. The distribution of each of the independent variable x and the dependent variable y (or the errors) is normal.
3. Variance is constant for each value of the independent variable.

The best approach to understand if these assumptions hold is to examine the residuals from the model. If all the assumptions hold, then the residual distribution will be *normal*, with *a mean of zero* and *constant variance* across the predicted-dependent variable (Fig. 9.4).

Below I show you how normally distributed residuals should look:

Residuals are distributed along the line. Their variance should not show any distribution patterns since they represent the *random component* of regression and therefore can't be predicted, as shown below (Fig. 9.5):

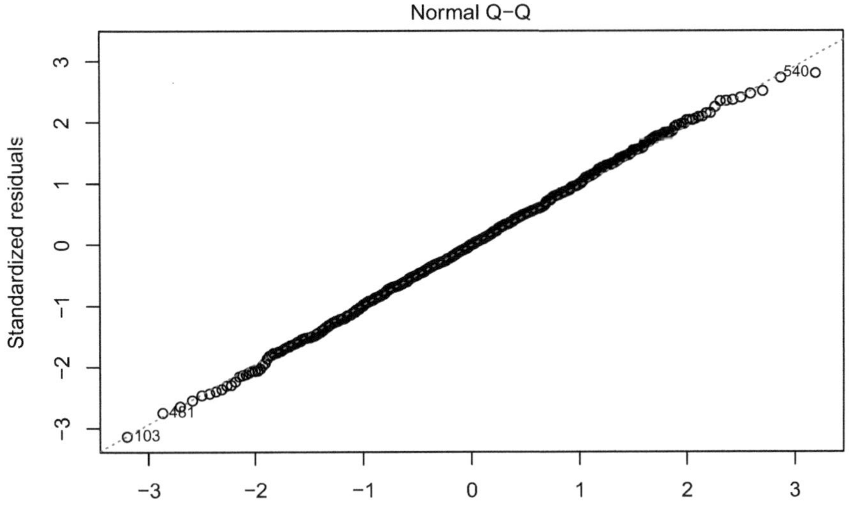

Fig. 9.4 Quantile-quantile plot with normally distributed residuals

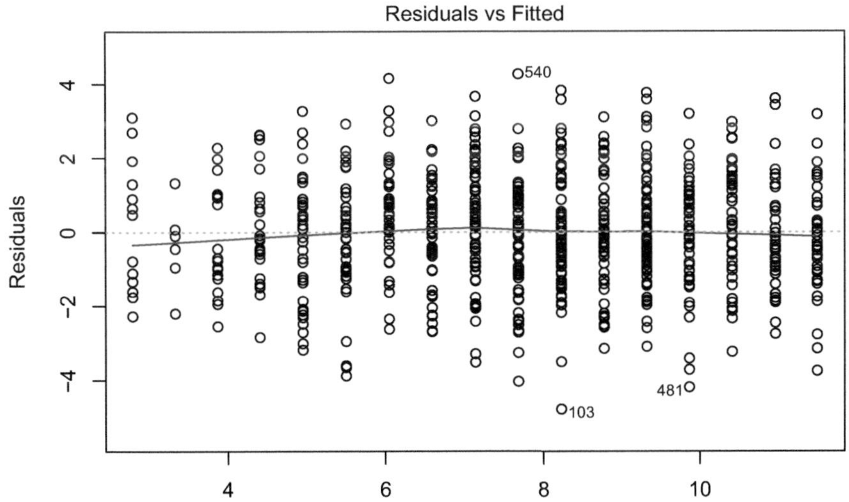

Fig. 9.5 Random distribution of the residuals with not organised patterns

We can now check the assumption in our simple linear regression model with some functions included in the `sjPlot` package.

```
> install.packages('sjPlot')
> library(sjPlot)
> plot_model(mymodel, type='diag')# we should specify that the
type should be = 'dig' as diagnostic.
```

The `plot_model` function returns some useful diagnostic plots. Here I use `type='diag'` to check if the assumptions hold (you should click on the arrows and scroll to see them all).

The first is the density distribution of the residuals with a normal distribution overlaid on the density distribution as shown below (Fig. 9.6):

From the plot in Fig. 9.6, the residual distribution looks fairly normally distributed (looks not dissimilar to the overlaid normal distribution).

Another informative plot is the quantile-quantile plot (Q-Q plot) (in the previous chapters, I introduced the normal distribution and how to check for normality, including the use of a Q-Q plot). The Q-Q plot is a plot of the quantiles of residuals,

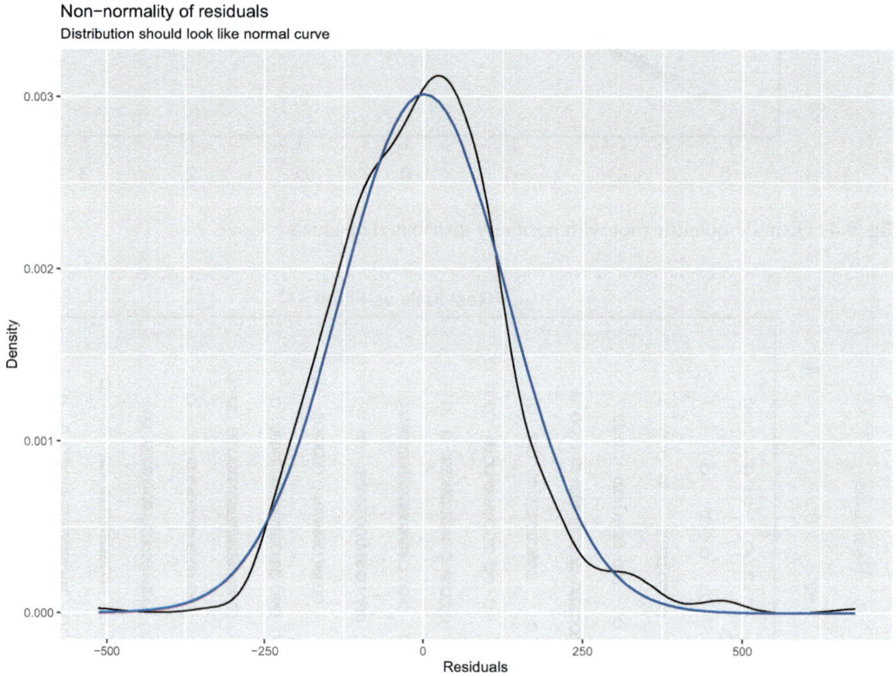

Fig. 9.6 Residual distribution with overlaid normal distribution

against the quantiles of the theoretical normal distribution. As I said, if the residuals are normally distributed, then the observations will lay on a straight line (Fig. 9.7):

From the Q-Q plot in Fig. 9.7, we can see many observations do not lie on the straight line. This is particularly true for the tails of the plot. You can see many *outliers* tailing off at the upper part of the Q-Q plot. This indicates that outliers may affect the regression model. This book covers the concept of outliers, high leverage and influential data points later in the book.

Nevertheless, you can expect to frequently see some drift in the tails of the distribution of a Q-Q plot, especially with a small sample size.

Moving forward, to assess the assumption of constant variance across the predictor, we should view the residuals by the fitted regression values, as shown in the plot in Fig. 9.8 (this is called *homoscedasticity*) (Fig. 9.8):

On this plot, the residuals are on the y-axis, and the fitted values from the regression line are on the x-axis. Ideally, we should expect equal scattering of the values above and below the mean with no recognisable or organised patterns of variability. In this specific case, however, there is evidence for non-constant variance (*heteroscedasticity*).

For the moment we can state that linear assumption may not hold, and we might consider to transform or manipulate the data to render the relationship linear. We will explore this later in this chapter

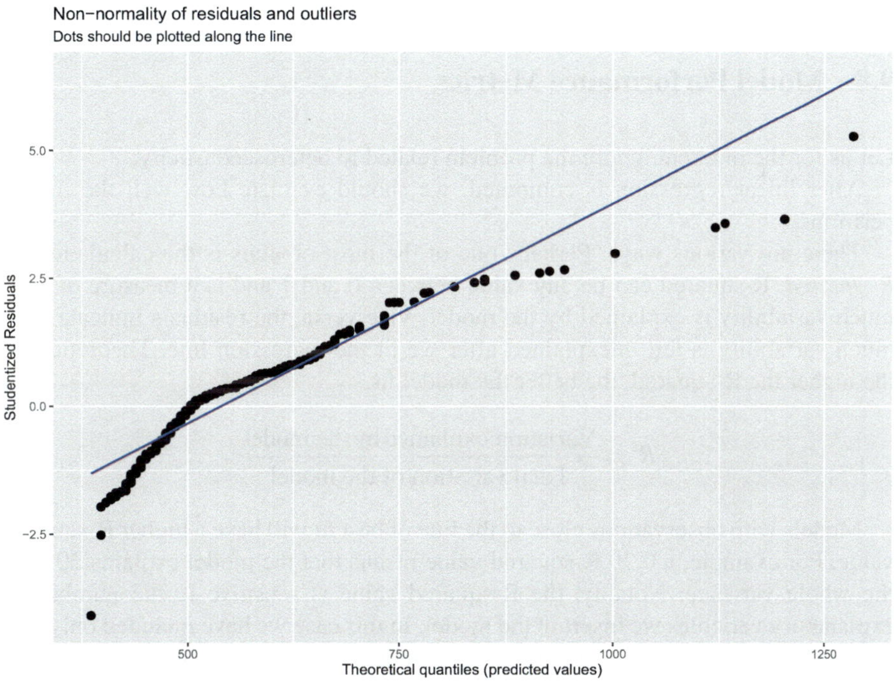

Fig. 9.7 Quantile-quantile residual plot showing asymmetry at the tails

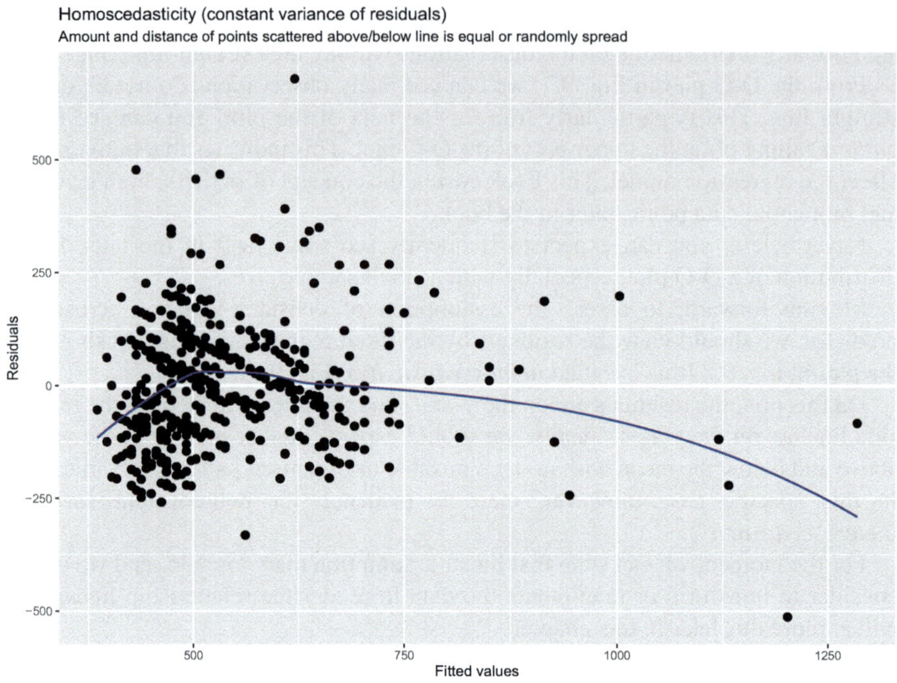

Fig. 9.8 Homoscedasticity

9.8 Model Performance Metrics

Let us for the moment ignore the problem related to heteroscedasticity.

After linear regression is computed, we should evaluate how well the model performs.

There are various ways. Perhaps one of the most obvious is the calculation of *R-squared*. R-squared can be any value between 0 and 1 and is a measure of how much variability is explained by the model. Vice versa, the residuals indicate how much variability is left unexplained after we fit the regression line. Theoretically, the higher the R-squared, the better the model fit.

$$R^2 = \frac{\text{Variation explained by the model}}{\text{Total variation of the model}}$$

Models with observations close to the line of best fit will have a higher R-squared value. For example, a 0.20 R-squared value means that the model explains 20% of the whole variance. Notably, the R-squared value is sensitive to the number of explanatory variables we insert in the model. In this case we have included only one explanatory variable (the `CC` time). Usually, models are more articulated with many explanatory variables, whereby the R-squared value will artificially increase as the number of explanatory variables increases.

```
Residual standard error: 132.5 on 498 degrees of freedom
Multiple R-squared:  0.4108,	Adjusted R-squared:  0.4096
F-statistic: 347.2 on 1 and 498 DF,  p-value: < 2.2e-16
```

Fig. 9.9 Linear regression analysis with R-squared and adjusted R-squared

We should then *correct* the R-squared value, adjusting it by the number of variables included (the adjusted R-squared value accounts for the number of predictor variables included in the model). "R" does this work for us. The R-squared value, along with the adjusted R-squared value, is included in the summary function (Fig. 9.9):

```
> mymodel<-lm(MMstat$Bleeding~MMstat$CC)
> summary(mymodel)
```

This is obviously not very interesting for a model with a single explanatory variable, but will be more so for complex models with several predictors.

R-squared and adjusted R-squared can be interpreted as a measure of *goodness of fit* (GOF). Different from R-squared, the adjusted R-squared increases only when the new variable in the model improves the fit. Also, the adjusted R-squared decreases when the term does not improve the model fit sufficiently.

Another measure of GOF is the *standard error of regression*. This measure tells us how far, on average, the data points are from the regression line, and uses the same unit of measure of the response variable. Generally, the aim is to obtain a low standard error of regression that ultimately decreases as R-squared increases.

The *Akaike information criterion* (AIC) is another common measure of performance. It was developed by the Japanese statistician Hirotugu Akaike in 1970. AIC penalises the inclusion of additional variables in the model by increasing the error, hence the lower the AIC the better. Note that AIC should be used essentially to compare the performance of two or more models. AICc is a version of AIC corrected for small sample size.

Other measures include the *Bayesian information criteria* (BIC), which is similar to AIC with a stronger penalty for including additional variables. There is also *Mallows Cp* which is another variant of AIC.

Finally, the *F-test of overall significance* compares the model that we specified to a model with no explanatory variable (the intercept model only). If none of the explanatory variables are significant, the overall F-test is also not significant. In our case the model returns a significant p-value and it means that our results likely did not happen by chance.

I have briefly mentioned GOF here; however, there is little point in scrutinising for goodness of fit in case of heteroscedasticity, when the linearity assumption does not hold. We will see some attempts to transform and manipulate data to address the non-linearity issue later in this chapter.

First, let's take a look at multivariable regression, where we will repeat the same statistical exercise in terms of assumption checking (residual evaluation) and goodness of fit.

9.9 Multivariable Linear Regression

Simple linear regression has a dependent variable, which is the outcome of interest, explained by a single independent variable, considered as the predictor. Adding more explanatory variables will transform the linear regression from simple to multivariable. Again, by definition, the dependent variables must be of a continuous structure. But importantly, the explanatory variables can be a combination of numeric, binary or ordinal. However, the interpretation of the β coefficient changes. Below is the formula for multivariable regression. We still have the intercept α and the random error ε. However, more explanatory variables $\beta_2 x_2 \ldots$ are also added:

$$y = \alpha + \beta_1 x_1 + \beta_2 x_2 \ldots + \varepsilon$$

Let us assume we want to model the continuous `Bleeding` variable with the binary `Broccoli` variable and the continuous numeric `CC` (cross-clamp) variable (Fig. 9.10):

```
> broccolimodel<-lm(MMstat$Bleeding~MMstat$Broccoli+MMstat$CC)
> summary(broccolimodel)
```

Note that the explanatory binary `Broccoli` variable has two levels, `y` and `n`. "R" automatically reads `'n'` as the reference level. Therefore, `Broccoli=='n'` is equal to zero and `Broccoli=='y'` is equal to 1.

The estimate associated to `Broccoliy` is −54.7. To understand its meaning, let us write the formula substituting the symbols with their respective values:

$$y = 334.29 - 54.47 * 1 \ldots + \beta 2x2$$

Let us omit for the moment $\beta 2$ which represents the coefficient associated to `CC`. The average bleeding (mL) in `Broccoliy` is 334.29 – 54.47*1=279.82. The intercept represents the mean bleeding when x equals zero. Since `Broccolin` was coded as equal to zero (reference level), the intercept represents the average bleeding in the no-broccoli group.

```
Coefficients:
                   Estimate Std. Error t value Pr(>|t|)
(Intercept)        334.2929    16.1624  20.683  < 2e-16 ***
MMstat$Broccoliy   -54.4740    12.2160  -4.459 1.02e-05 ***
MMstat$CC            5.5252     0.3192  17.310  < 2e-16 ***
---
Signif. codes:  0 '***' 0.001 '**' 0.01 '*' 0.05 '.' 0.1 ' ' 1
```

Fig. 9.10 Coefficient for the regression model

Let us complete the above formula by adding the CC estimates:

$$y = 334.29 - 54.47 * 1 + 5.52 * 1$$

Keeping constant $\beta 2$ as 1 minute (that is the unit of measure for CC), the average bleeding for the broccoli group would be 285.34 mL.

If dependency between β coefficient is noted, this phenomenon is called collinearity or multicollinearity, which is explained in greater detail in a dedicated paragraph later in this chapter.

9.10 Broccoli as a Factor or a Number?

Broccoli was coded as 'y' and 'n' and is clearly a factor. "R" assigned 'n' as the reference level (Broccolin = 0), because in the alphabet n comes first. Sometimes we want to code a factor to 0 and 1 for the sake of simplicity:

```
>  MMstat$Broccoli<-ifelse(test=MMstat$Broccoli=='y',   yes='1',
no='0')#using the function ifelse
> table(MMstat$Broccoli)
  0   1
297 203
> MMstat$Broccoli<-as.factor(MMstat$Broccoli)# converting Broccoli
0/1 to factor
```

However, the regression output (Fig. 9.11) remains the same for Broccoli1 and Broccoliy

```
Coefficients:
                 Estimate Std. Error t value Pr(>|t|)
(Intercept)       581.700      9.544  60.947  < 2e-16 ***
MMstat$Broccoli1 -106.321     14.979  -7.098 4.38e-12 ***
```

```
Coefficients:
                 Estimate Std. Error t value Pr(>|t|)
(Intercept)       581.700      9.544  60.947  < 2e-16 ***
MMstat$Broccoliy -106.321     14.979  -7.098 4.38e-12 ***
```

Fig. 9.11 Regression summary after converting Broccoli to number and to factor again

9.11 Adding Ordinal Variables with More than Two Levels

In the previous section we dealt with the binary `Broccoli` variable. The reference level was `Broccoli=='n'`. Hence, the beta coefficient was computed for `Broccoliy` keeping `Broccolin` as the reference. In a context of β equals zero, the intercept represents the average bleeding for `Broccoli=='n'`.

But what if the explanatory variable is ordinal with many levels?

As an example, in the `MMstat` dataset we have the `Diabetes` variable which has three levels (0=no diabetes, 1=non-insulin dependent, 2=insulin-dependent diabetes mellitus). What happens if we code to create a model for this variable? Below I run a simple regression model for brevity:

```
> MMstat$Diabetes<-as.factor(MMstat$Diabetes)
> myordinalmodel<-lm(MMstat$Bleeding~MMstat$Diabetes)
> summary(myordinalmodel)
```

The model returns the beta factors of levels `MMstat$Diabetes1` and `MMstat$Diabetes2` keeping level 0 as the reference (i.e. `MMstat$Diabetes0`) (Fig. 9.12):

The average of `Bleeding` (y) = 534.77 (α)+45.66 (β for `MMstat$Diabetes2`) + random error ε, while keeping in mind the output is in comparison to `MMstat$Diabetes0`.

It seems that having insulin-dependent diabetes increases average bleeding by 45.66 mL, when compared to those with no diabetes. However, we cannot reject the null hypothesis since the p-value is high at a significant level of .05.

It is possible to change the reference level. With the `relevel( )` function and `ref=2` argument as follows (Fig. 9.13):

```
Coefficients:
                  Estimate Std. Error t value Pr(>|t|)
(Intercept)        534.777      8.489  62.997   <2e-16 ***
MMstat$Diabetes1    16.166     22.164   0.729    0.466
MMstat$Diabetes2    45.660     43.956   1.039    0.299
```

Fig. 9.12 Linear regression with ordinal Diabetes variable where no diabetes (level = 0) is the reference

```
Coefficients:
                  Estimate Std. Error t value Pr(>|t|)
(Intercept)         550.94      20.47  26.910   <2e-16 ***
MMstat$Diabetes0    -16.17      22.16  -0.729    0.466
MMstat$Diabetes2     29.49      47.74   0.618    0.537
```

Fig. 9.13 Changing the reference level for ordinal variables

```
> MMstat$Diabetes<-relevel(MMstat$Diabetes, ref=2)# in this case
we set the reference level as MMstat$Diabetes2
> mymodelR<-lm(MMstat$Bleeding~MMstat$Diabetes)
> summary(mymodelR)
```

As per the output above, the reference level is level 2, which corresponds to insulin-dependent diabetes mellitus (0 = no diabetes, 1= non-insulin dependent, 2 = insulin-dependent diabetes mellitus). You may notice that the sign of the `MMstat$Diabetes0` beta coefficient is now negative, indicating a reduction in the average bleeding.

9.12 Collinearity

A multivariable model is based, by definition, on more than one explanatory term. However, by the time we include terms in the model, we may run into some issues. One of them is collinearity.

The lack of change in most of the coefficients between the simple model and the multivariable model should reassure you that collinearity is unlikely to be a problem in the model. But what is collinearity? It occurs when there are high correlations amongst explanatory variables, leading to unstable regression coefficients. This means that an independent variable can be predicted from another in the regression model. For example, height and weight can be two variables affected by collinearity. This is an example of structural multicollinearity because usually taller people weigh more. We assume collinearity between those two variables, where we cannot partition the variance between the two, and evaluate the effect on the dependent variable.

Another example may be the redundant coding with a *dummy variable*. This is very common in medicine. For example, let us assume that I recorded the left ventricle function on a scale from 10% to 70%. I also coded in another column the same left ventricle function in an ordinal scale (10–30 = poor, 30–50=moderate, >50=good). This is an example of artificial collinearity, also named as data multicollinearity. Those variables are redundant and can inflate the system since they are highly correlated. It would also be difficult to separate the effect of each other on the outcome of interest.

Multicollinearity is a common problem when estimating linear and generalised linear models including Cox regression.

The most widely used diagnostic for collinearity is the variance inflation factor (*VIF*). It is named variance inflation since it estimates how much the variance of a coefficient is *inflated* because of linear dependence of other predictors.

VIF has a lower bound of 1 with no upper limit. A VIF of 1.6 means that the variance of that particular coefficient is 60% larger than it would be if that predictor was completely non-correlated to the others. To check for collinearity, we can use the `rms` package. As before, we use the `vif` function specifying `type='diag'`.

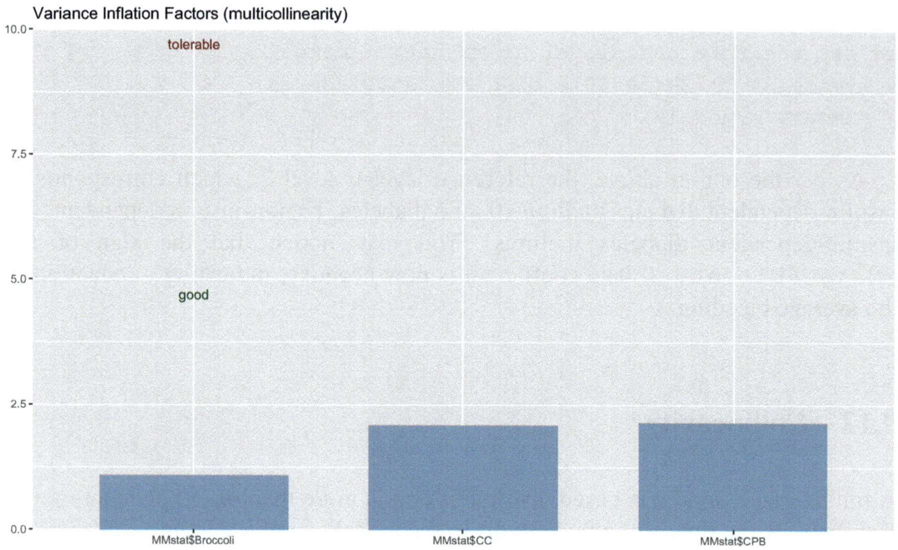

Fig. 9.14 Variance inflation factors

Let us consider the following model (Fig. 9.14):

```
> library(rms)#we need this library
>  vifmodel<-lm(MMstat$Bleeding~MMstat$Broccoli+MMstat$CC+MMstat$
CPB)
> vif(vifmodel) #using the function vif
MMstat$Broccoliy          MMstat$CC        MMstat$CPB
        1.094733           2.090240          2.144196
> plot_model(vifmodel, type='diag')
```

Generally, a VIF lower than 5 does not affect the beta regression coefficient (the green dotted line in the plot in Fig. 9.14). As you can see from Fig. 9.14, in our reduced model, composed of three explanatory variables, no significant VIF was detected.

Multicollinearity weakens the statistical power of the regression model and the coefficients become very sensitive to small changes in the model.

9.13 Interaction

While building our model with many terms, another issue to be aware of is *interaction*.

The *main effect* is the portion of the effect of a certain explanatory variable x on the response variable y that does not depend on the values of the other variables in the model.

The *interaction effect* (also called *effect modification*) indicates a portion of the effect of an explanatory variable x that depends on the value of at least one other independent variable x_n in the model.

In fact, interaction effect indicates that a *third variable* influences the relationship between the independent and dependent variables.

As an example, say we want to examine the effect of operation time on bleeding. However other variables, such as taking an antiplatelet agent like aspirin, may *interact* with the operation time variable and create an effect modification.

Age, race and gender are generally common explanatory variables that may show a degree of interaction with a certain response variable.

We should be very well aware of interaction terms in regression, since they can be crucial in the model building/interpretation process.

The regression model for interaction is computed as per the formula:

$$y = \alpha + \beta_1 x_1 + \beta_2 x_2 + \beta_3 x_1 * x_2 \ldots + \varepsilon$$

Included in the regression model is the two-way effect modification:

$$\beta_3 x_1 * x_2$$

How to detect interaction $x_1 * x_2 - > y$?

An *interaction plot* is a way to detect potential interaction effect amongst variables.

Let us assume that we want to explore (i.e. to include in the model) a plausible interaction between ischaemic time `CC`, cardio-pulmonary bypass `CPB`, `Aspirin` and `Broccoli`. In this case we must explore potential interaction between numeric and binomial explanatory variables.

The operator for interaction is either the star symbol `*` or the colon `:`.

First, we explore the interaction terms for each couple separately, then plot them together using the `gridExtra` library (Fig. 9.15):

```
> intermodel1<-lm(Bleeding~CC*Aspirin, data=MMstat)
a<-plot_model(intermodel1, type='int') #no interaction
> intermodel2<-lm(Bleeding~CPB*Aspirin, data=MMstat)
> b<-plot_model(intermodel2, type='int')#yes interaction
> intermodel3<-lm(Bleeding~CPB*Broccoli, data=MMstat)
> c<-plot_model(intermodel3, type='int')#no interaction
> intermodel4<-lm(Bleeding~CC*Broccoli, data=MMstat)
> d<-plot_model(intermodel4, type='int')#yes interaction

grid.arrange(a,b,c,d)
```

As you can see from Fig. 9.14, there might be an interaction between `Aspirin` and `CPB` and between `Broccoli` and `CC` on the panels to the right.

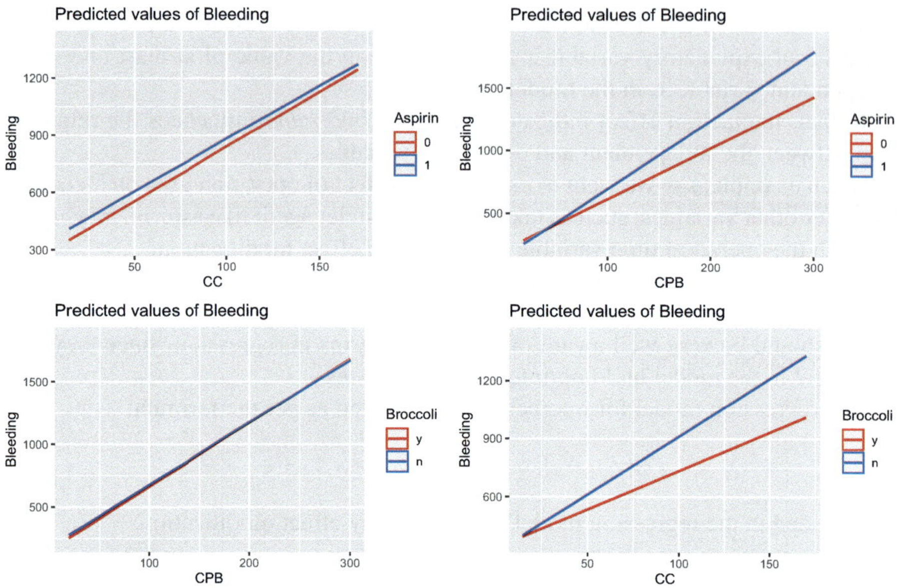

Fig. 9.15 Interaction analysis

```
Coefficients:
              Estimate Std. Error t value Pr(>|t|)
(Intercept)   313.1883    17.8678  17.528  < 2e-16 ***
CC              5.9965     0.3622  16.556  < 2e-16 ***
Broccoliy      21.5381    30.6991   0.702  0.48327
CC:Broccoliy   -2.0226     0.7503  -2.696  0.00726 **
```

Fig. 9.16 Linear regression summary showing the estimate for the interaction between two variables (cross-clamp and Broccoli)

In general, if the lines on the interaction plot are parallel, then there is no interaction effect. Vice versa if the lines are not parallel and intersect, there is likely an interaction effect. The more non-parallel the lines are, the greater the strength of the interaction.

If, for example, we use the `summary( )` function for `intermodel4`, we see that the interaction term is statistically significant (Fig. 9.16):

When an interaction effect is significant, we should not interpret the isolated effect of the variables (the *main effect*). However, the question remains: should we include the significant interaction in the model? The answer is yes, if it makes sense conceptually. In fact, in order to include interaction in the model, it must be both statistically significant and conceptually viable. Do consider that the `lm( )` function does not include interaction terms per se. We must specifically add what we believe is important logically and conceptually to the model.

9.14 Model Building Strategy

We have reached the stage where we should think about which explanatory variables to include in the model and how to address the non-linearity issue given the non-normal distribution of the residuals. Our MMstat dataset contains many unusual observations. Some of them may be data entry errors, or they may be *real* observations which are simply unusual.

In an ideal world, we should aim for a model with no overfitting that is also simple. Consider a more parsimonious model is always preferable, with a high adjusted R-squared and a low standard error of regression as a measure of GOF. Obviously, for this hypothetical model, the linearity assumption must hold, along with normal distribution of the residuals. When we refer to normal distribution, we refer to the *residual error* distribution rather than the dependent or independent variables. Those variables may not be normally distributed and yet have a linear relationship. Again, we should understand whether the residuals are normally distributed rather than investigating normality distribution at the level of the response or explanatory variables.

Nevertheless, variables with Gaussian distribution can be more prone to a linear relationship, which is why data transformation (e.g. log/Box-Cox...) is often advisable.

Also, we should keep in mind that unusual observations, or outliers, may have a *leverage effect* on both the performance of the prediction and the effect size model.

9.15 Including the Variables of Interest

Our MMstat dataset contains 12 potential pre-operative explanatory variables (excluding ID) that may affect the Bleeding response variable:

```
> names(MMstat)
 [1] "ID"          "Age"          "Male"
 [4] "Weight"      "Height"       "Diabetes"
 [7] "COPD"        "LVEF"         "Creatinine"
[10] "Aspirin"     "Broccoli"     "CPB"
[13] "CC"
```

Some of these variables can be correlated. In the chapter about correlation (specifically in the correlation matrix section), I demonstrated (as expected) that Weight and Height are correlated. Therefore, to simplify the model, we can calculate body mass index and add a column in the dataset:

```
> bmi<-MMstat$Weight/(MMstat$Height/100)^2# bmi formula = weight/
kilogram^2
> MMstat$bmi<-bmi # adding the bmi to MMstat
```

By doing so, we have started simplifying the model.

Another consideration examines CC and CPB. From a numerical point of view, even if the VIF analysis did not detect significant collinearity, those variables are in fact correlated. Also, from a conceptual point of view, the ischaemic time (CC) is a surgical momentum that occurs during the cardio-pulmonary bypass (CPB). With this in mind we can advance the hypothesis to drop the CC variable since it might be conceptually included in the CPB variable.

Rather than performing a statistical pre-screening, for example, including only variables that are significant at *bivariate analysis level*, we should include all elements that theoretically we know from previous research/experience/literature may affect the response.

After simplification, the explanatory variables which I believe may model the response variable follow (Fig. 9.17):

```
> analysisfull<-lm(Bleeding~Broccoli+CPB+Age+Male+Diabetes+Aspiri
n+Creatinine+COPD+ LVEF+bmi, data=MMstat)
> summary(analysisfull)
```

And the confint( ) function returns the 95% CI (Fig. 9.18):

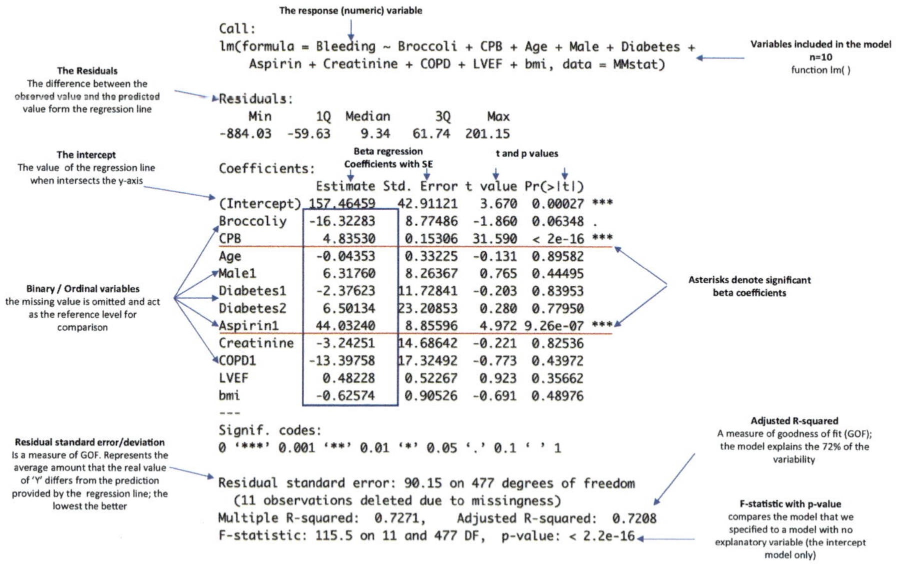

Fig. 9.17 Full summary of the linear regression model

Fig. 9.18 95% confidence interval of the estimate from the regression model

	2.5 %	97.5 %
(Intercept)	73.1462143	241.7829638
Broccoliy	-33.5650010	0.9193360
CPB	4.5345382	5.1360628
Age	-0.6963785	0.6093221
Male1	-9.9201013	22.5552960
Diabetes1	-25.4219764	20.6695124
Diabetes2	-39.1022586	52.1049380
Aspirin1	26.6308762	61.4339255
Creatinine	-32.1005925	25.6155719
COPD1	-47.4401856	20.6450194
LVEF	-0.5447461	1.5093132
bmi	-2.4045304	1.1530474

```
> confint(analysisfull)
```

Note that for `CPB` and `Aspirin` the 95% CI does not include zero; hence, the value is significant. How to interpret the beta coefficient? In this example, the coefficient for `CPB` is 4.8. This means when keeping all the other variables constant, each minute `CPB` increases, the average bleeding increases by 4.8 mL. When considering the `Aspirin` variable, the average increase is 26.6 *1 (1= `Aspirin` / 0= `no Aspirin`). Note the `Broccoli` variable has an almost significant p-value. The R-squared in its adjusted form is acceptable, explaining the 72% variability of the model, along with the F-test statistic which has a significant p-value, suggesting a good model performance. Finally, note that the beta coefficients have to be interpreted as adjusted given the multivariable regression model constructed. At this stage, no interaction terms were included.

Before jumping to final conclusions saying that `CPB` and `Aspirin` are independent predictors for post-operative bleeding, we should check the distribution of the residuals to assess if the linearity assumption holds.

9.16 Model Diagnostic

As explained before I should run a model diagnostic test as below (Fig. 9.19):

```
> plot_model(analysisfull, type='diag')
```

A significant non-normal distribution in the residual is noted since they do not overlap the plotted blue line and significantly tail off. With this in mind, linearity assumptions do not hold and we should address this non-linearity to proceed. It is always advisable to use the function `?` to ask for help. For example,

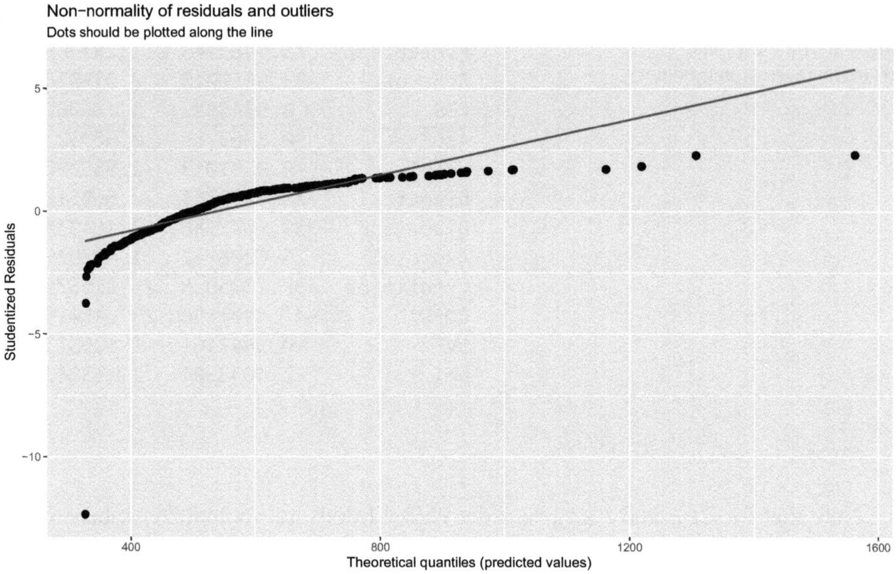

Fig. 9.19 Diagnostic plot

```
>?plot_model
```

returns the help menu for the `plot_model` function, from the `sjPlot` package. I also specify the `type='diag'` *diagnostic* function since I would like to run a diagnostic test.

9.17 Addressing Non-linearity

The model we have selected has some non-linearity issues. Before interpreting the results, we must overcome this problem.

There are some potential methods to address the non-linearity issue if we would like to stick to non-linear terms. Below I discuss those which represent the most popular ones:

1. Transform *y* using `log(y)` or the squared root of *y*. `log` can address the heteroscedasticity (the non-constant variance, since the variability in y is reduced). However, for an effective model, we may lose interpretability. It works better for predictive purposes. Here is the code with the `log(Bleeding)` function highlighted in red:

```
> analysisfull<-lm(log(Bleeding)~Broccoli+CPB+Age+Male
+Diabetes+Aspirin+Creatinine+COPD+ LVEF+bmi, data=MMstat)
```

2. Transform x in the same way as y. We may want to focus on Gaussian distribution. The quality and reliability of linear regression might depend also on the underlying variables' distributions. The model will return more reliable predictions if dependent and independent variables have Gaussian distribution:

```
> analysisfull<-lm(log(Bleeding)~Broccoli+log(CPB)+log
(Age)+Male+Diabetes+Aspirin+                              log
(Creatinine)+COPD+log(LVEF)+log(bmi),data=MMstat)
```

   By doing this, I apply `log` transformation to all the numeric variables in the scenario.
3. Polynomial terms/quadratic: X^2 (additional inflection). It fits a more natural scenario. *Polynomial regression* is a special case of linear regression where the relationship between x and y is modelled using a *polynomial*, rather than a *line*.

   It might be used in the context of non-linearity. Polynomial is still considered a particular case of multiple linear regression. For the sake of clarity, I provide an example of a simple regression below (Fig. 9.20):

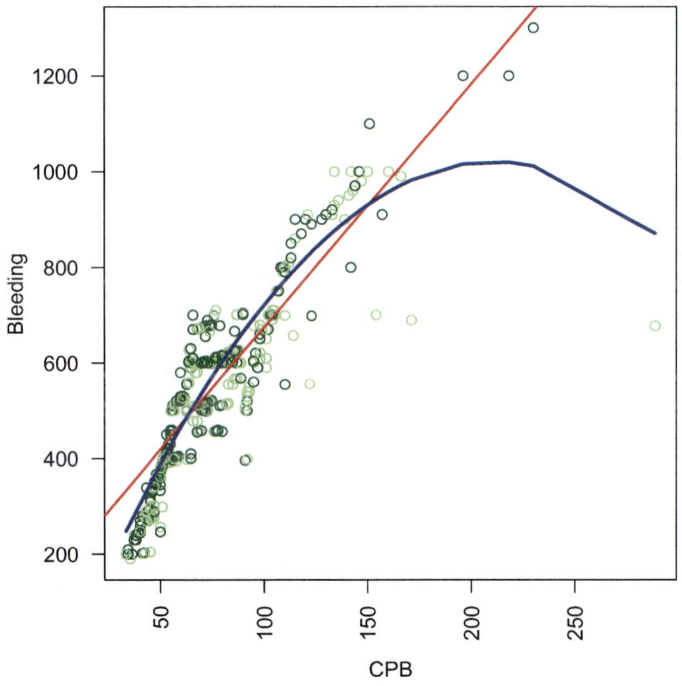

Fig. 9.20 Polynomial regression analysis

```
> plot(CPB, Bleeding, las=2, col=c('darkgreen',
'lightgreen'))#attached MMstat
> lineanalysis<-lm(Bleeding~CPB)
> abline(lineanalysis, col='red', lwd=2)
> polyanalysis<-lm(Bleeding~poly(CPB, degree = 2, raw=T))
#similar to
> polyanalysis<-lm(Bleeding~CPB+I(CPB^2))
> lines(smooth.spline(CPB, predict(polyanalysis)),
col='blue', lwd=3)
```

To apply polynomial (in this case for the variable `CPB`) we should use the code `CPB+I(CPB^2)`, with the function `I`, and square the variable. Importantly the variable `CPB` should also be left unsquared as `CPB+I(CPB^2)` and included in the analysis.

The figure above reproduces the two regression lines. The *red line* equals the linear regression model and the *blue line* equals the polynomial regression model.

The downside of the model is that we may lose interpretability.

We can also try to fit a cubic analysis and compare the two models with the `anova( )` function (Fig. 9.21):

```
> cubeanalysis<-lm(Bleeding~CPB+I(CPB^2)+I(CPB^3))
> anova(polyanalysis,cubeanalysis)
```

As set out in the figure above, `anova` returns a non-significant p-value, suggesting no differences between the two models. In essence, the cubic term does not improve the model.

4. Box-Cox transformation of the *y* response variable. A Box-Cox (from the names of the two statisticians who theorised the transformation) is a transformation of non-normal dependent variables into a normal shape. At the base of the Box-Cox transformation is an exponent, lambda (λ), which works well from −3 to 3. The *optimal λ value* is the one which results in the best approximation of a normal distribution curve. The function to use is `boxcox( )` (Fig. 9.22):

```
Analysis of Variance Table

Model 1: Bleeding ~ CPB + I(CPB^2)
Model 2: Bleeding ~ CPB + I(CPB^2) + I(CPB^3)
  Res.Df     RSS Df Sum of Sq      F Pr(>F)
1    497 2951324
2    496 2951124  1    200.57 0.0337 0.8544
```

Fig. 9.21 Anova analysis of two polynomial models

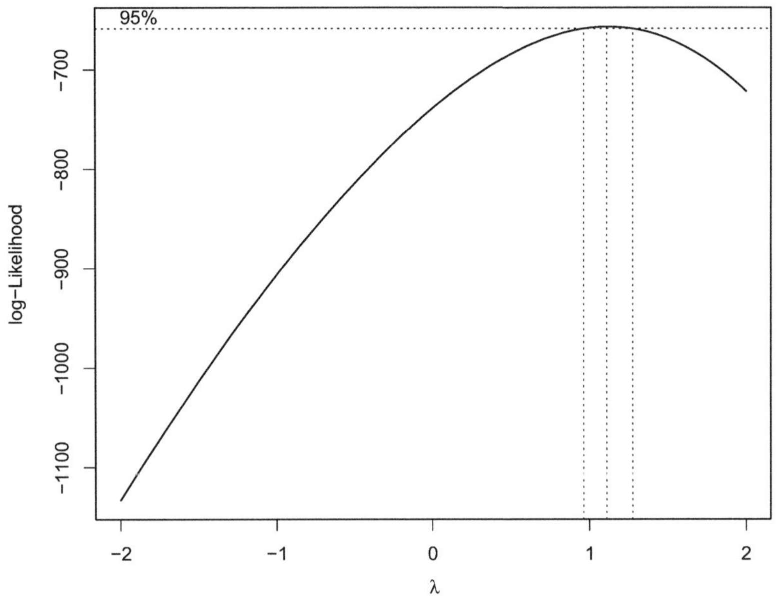

Fig. 9.22 Box-Cox transformation with optimal lambda

```
> attach(MMstat)
> library(MASS)
> bc<-boxcox(Bleeding~Broccoli+CPB+Age+Male+Diabetes+A
spirin+Creatinine+COPD+LVEF+bmi, data=MMstat)
> lambda <- bc$x[which.max(bc$y)]
> lambda
[1] 1.1
```

In the figure above, the dotted lines indicate the 95% CI around the lambda. The best lambda in our case is +1.11. We should then add it to the model:

```
> new_model <- lm(((Bleeding^lambda-1)/lambda) ~ Brocc
oli+CPB+Age+Male+Diabetes+Aspirin+Creatinine+COPD+LVEF+bmi,
data=MMstat)
```

Notably, Box-Cox only works if *y* contains all positive values. Applying Box-Cox transformation for the *x* variables is uncommon (*but not impossible*). Nevertheless, the vast majority of Box-Cox transformation is only applied to the response variable. Here I perform a diagnostic, this time using the basic `plot(new_model)` function (Fig. 9.23):

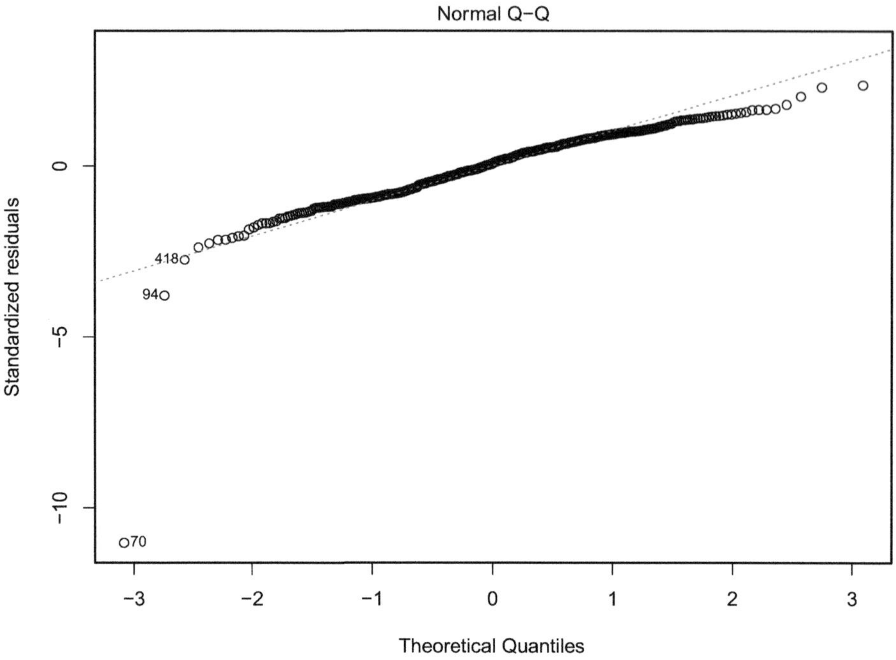

Fig. 9.23 Quantile-quantile residuals plot after Box-Cox transformation

```
> plot(new_model)# This time I used the basic function
'plot' to check the model. I could also use the function plot_
model(new_model, type= 'diag'), from the package sjPlot as pre-
viously carried out.
Hit <Return> to see next plot:
```

In the figure above, you may notice that the distribution of the residuals is more accurate, since we gained some degree of *normality*. However, outliers may still affect the system as shown in both tails of the Q-Q plot.

The figure below sets out the model summary after Box-Cox transformation of the dependent variable (Fig. 9.24):

Notably after transformation, the explanatory variable of the `Broccoli` interest is now associated to a significant p-value.

5. Removing outliers. We should always be aware of *noise*. Linear regression can be affected by *noisy/unusual* observations. Outliers, being unusual observations, may affect the line of linear regression analysis. Outliers or unusual observations can simply be data error entries or real atypical observations. Sometimes outliers may not affect the linear model at all and vice versa can be very informative. Sometimes it is more important to remove outliers with regard to the output/dependent variable.

```
Coefficients:
             Estimate Std. Error t value Pr(>|t|)
(Intercept) 203.93448   85.64036   2.381   0.0176 *
Broccoliy   -34.59067   17.51250  -1.975   0.0488 *
CPB           9.85043    0.30548  32.246  < 2e-16 ***
Age           0.05791    0.66309   0.087   0.9304
Male1        12.92909   16.49228   0.784   0.4335
Diabetes1    -5.95746   23.40707  -0.255   0.7992
Diabetes2    12.02123   46.31859   0.260   0.7953
Aspirin1     86.78933   17.67435   4.910 1.25e-06 ***
Creatinine   -5.76339   29.31053  -0.197   0.8442
COPD1       -30.90811   34.57634  -0.894   0.3718
LVEF          0.90093    1.04313   0.864   0.3882
bmi          -1.39882    1.80668  -0.774   0.4392
---
Signif. codes:  0 '***' 0.001 '**' 0.01 '*' 0.05 '.' 0.1 ' ' 1
```

Fig. 9.24 Summary after Box-Cox transformation

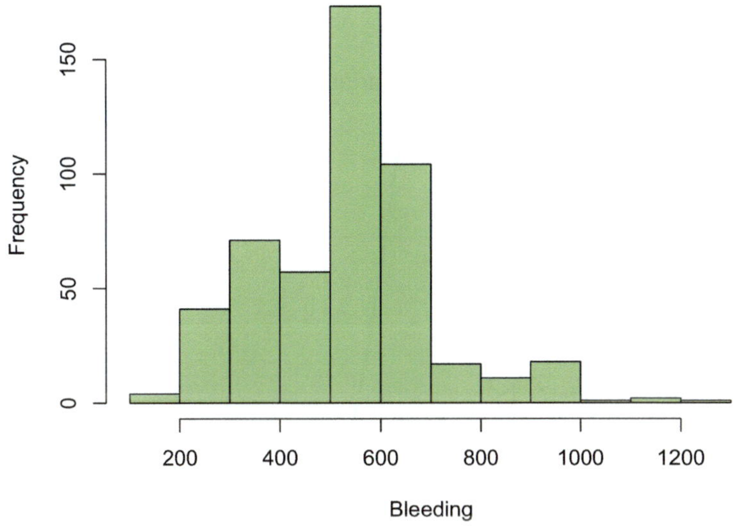

Fig. 9.25 Histogram and outlier detection

The decision whether to remove or keep outliers should be preceded by an in-depth clinical evaluation.

Below I provide an example on how to remove outliers from the `Bleeding` response variable. To do so we should first plot the observations to identify the outliers (Fig. 9.25):

```
> hist(MMstat$Bleeding, col='lightgreen', xlab='Bleeding',
main='Bleeding')
```

As you can see in the figure above, many unusual observations are located on the right side of the plot (right skewed distribution). Let us have a look at the density plot (Fig. 9.26):

```
> ggdensity(MMstat$Bleeding, main = "Density plot of
response variable Bleeding", xlab = "Bleeding ml",
col='darkgreen', lwd=1)
```

By analysing the plots in Figs. 9.24 and 9.25, we may want to consider the option to remove outliers above 800 mL, assigning `<-NA` to all observations above 800:

```
> MMstat$Bleeding[MMstat$Bleeding>800]<-NA
```

This is how the distribution looks after removing the right tailed outliers (Fig. 9.27):

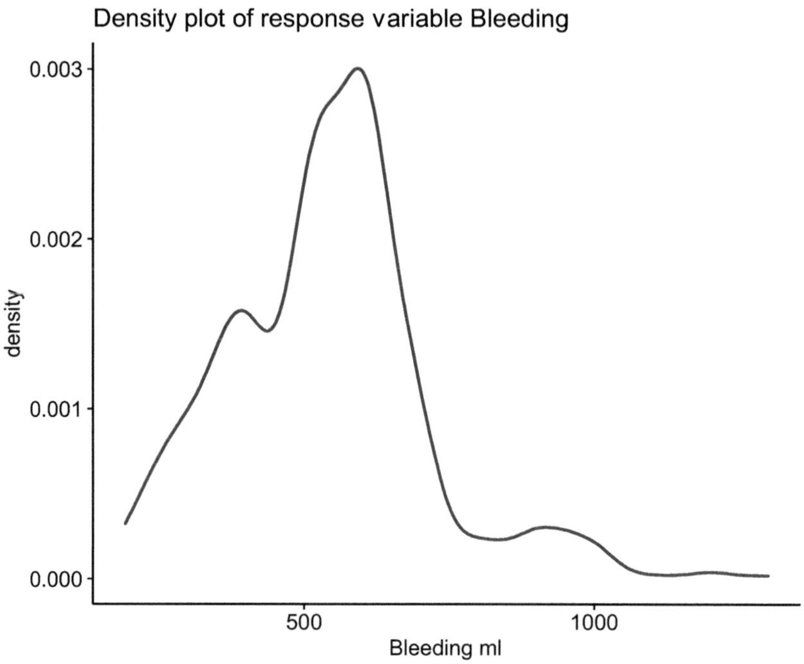

Fig. 9.26 Density plot and outlier detection

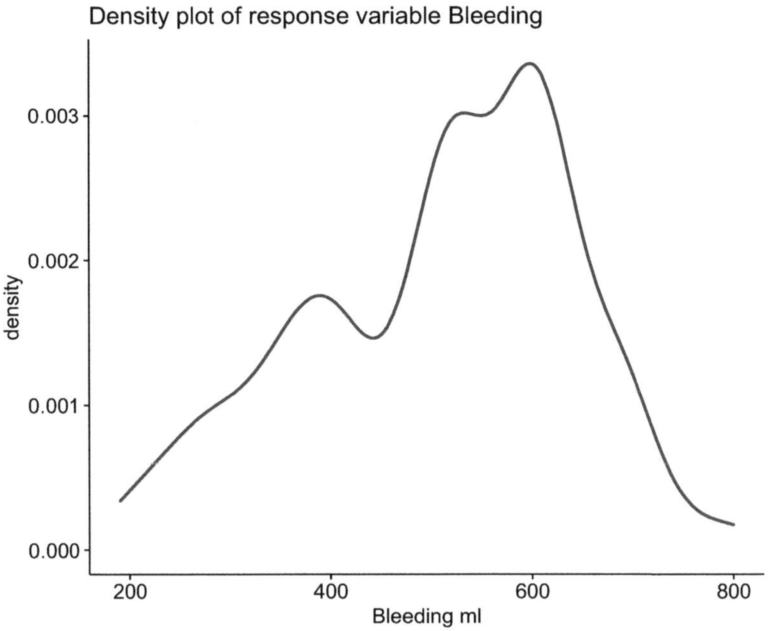

Fig. 9.27 Density plot after excluding outliers

6. Addressing collinearity. Linear regression will overfit your data when you have highly correlated input variables with no possibility to partition variance amongst explanatory variables. To address this, you must identify the most correlated variables with variance inflation analysis and consider removing the most correlated. Below I use the `plot_model(analysisfull, type='diag')` function (Fig. 9.28):

```
> analysisfull<-lm(Bleeding~Broccoli+CPB+Age+Male+Diab
etes+Aspirin+Creatinine+COPD+
LVEF+bmi, data=MMstat)
> plot_model(analysisfull, type='diag')
```

We have already addressed some data and structural collinearity (i.e. `weight` and `height` which were transformed to `bmi`, and `CPB` and `CC` where the latter was excluded). Now we calculate the VIF, yet none of the explanatory variables included seem to show significant signs of collinearity.

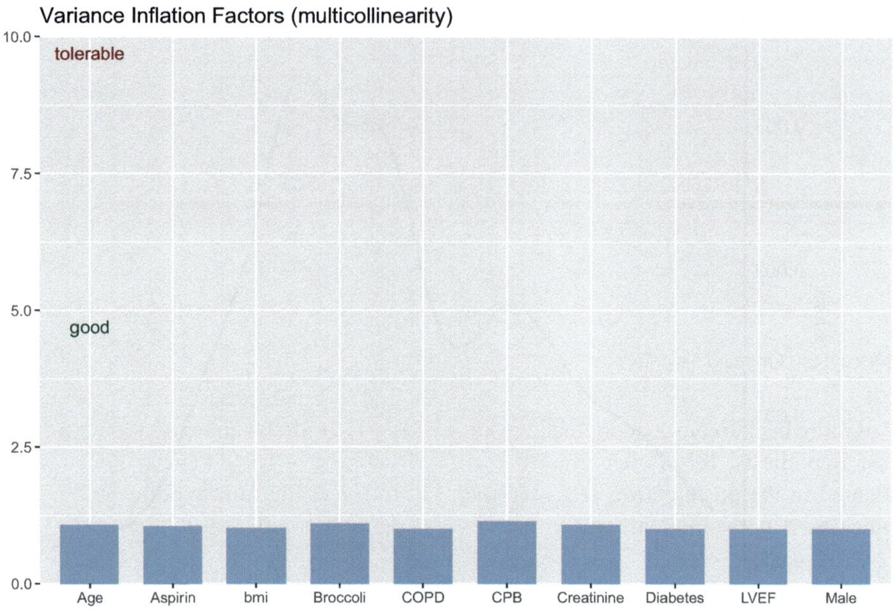

Fig. 9.28 Variance inflation factor to detect potential collinearity

9.18 Influential Data Points

Outliers are data points that stand out from the others and have unusual values on the y-axis, hence high residual values. *High leverage* data points are unusual points on the x-axis. The latter represents extreme values on the x-axis, yet they remain following the same direction of the line of best fit. When data points have both high residuals (outliers) and extreme values on the x-axis (high leverage), they are likely to influence the regression output, hence categorised as *influential observations*. The best way to detect an influential observation is by calculating the Cook's distance. This topic is also covered in the chapter on logistic regression. For the time being I make an example of how to identify an influential observation and how to handle it.

Let us consider a simple model (Fig. 9.29):

```
> model<-lm(Bleeding~CPB, data=MMstat)
>       ggplot(MMstat,aes(CPB,       Bleeding))+geom_point()+geom_
smooth(method = 'lm', se=FALSE)+ggtitle('A')
```

From Fig. 9.29a, it is intuitive to detect an unusual observation on the right side of the picture (the squared data point). This observation has both extreme x-values and high residuals. The Cook's distance will help us to identify the unusual observation (Fig. 9.30):

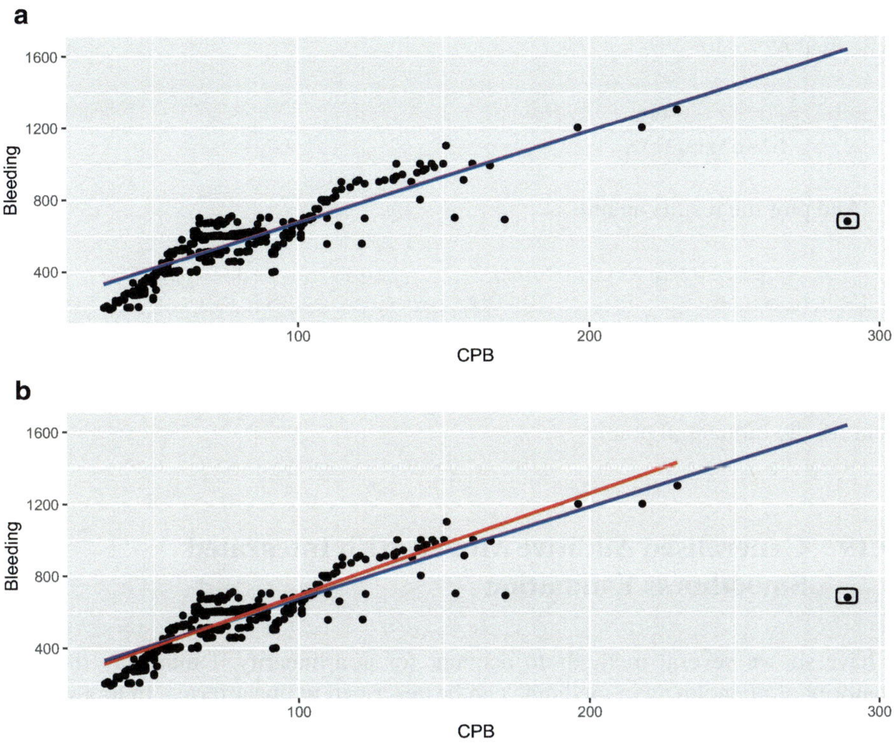

Fig. 9.29 Detecting unusual observation. Regression line (**a**) before and (**b**) after removing influential points

Fig. 9.30 Cook's distance to identify the influential data point. Generally, a Cook's D above 1 represents an influential data point

```
# A tibble: 6 × 3
  Bleeding   CPB cooks_dist
     <int> <int>      <dbl>
1      677   289     8.05
2      689   171     0.190
3      700   154     0.0682
4     1100   151     0.0280
5      556   122     0.0248
6     1200   218     0.0201
```

```
> cooks.distance(model)
model %>%
  augment %>%
  dplyr::select(Bleeding, CPB,cooks_dist=.cooksd) %>%
  arrange(desc(cooks_dist)) %>%
  head()
```

In this case, we should remove the variable that corresponds to the individual who bled 677 mL:

```
> newbleeding<-MMstat %>%
  filter(Bleeding!=677)
```

And plot the results again:

```
>      ggplot(MMstat,aes(CPB,      Bleeding))+geom_point()+geom_
smooth(method  =  'lm',  se=FALSE)+geom_smooth(method  =  'lm',
se=FALSE, data=newbleeding, col='red')+ggtitle('B')
```

In Fig. 9.29b you can see how the regression line (in red) changes after we remove the influential point.

9.19 Generalised Additive Models with Integrated Smoothness Estimation

I have shown several methods to account for non-linearity. I must say the vast majority of phenomena in medicine can be described in linear terms. In this section I touch upon non-linear models. Nevertheless, I will only scratch the surface, since in-depth description of non-linear models goes beyond the scope of this book.

Perhaps, given the nature of our data, another plausible approach would be to accept components of non-linearity of the model since we may believe that non-linear terms may also explain the relationship between dependent and independent variables. This is where generalised additive models are useful.

Generalised additive models (GAMs) can fit complex non-linear relationship phenomenon using a *smooth* or *spline function* `s( )` for any numerical variables which we believe would be best described with non-linear terms.

Multivariable GAMs accommodate continuous and non-numeric explanatory variables, with the possibility to combine linear and non-linear relationships. When categorical variables (linear term) are included in the model, GAM returns a fix effect for each level of the categories. GAMs are very flexible. Nevertheless, flexibility comes at a cost, with less interpretability given in the non-linear component of the model.

We use the `gam( )` function from the `mgcv` package:

```
> modelgam<-gam(Bleeding~Broccoli+s(CPB)+s(Age)+Male+Diabetes+Asp
irin+s(Creatinine)
+COPD+s(LVEF)+s(bmi), data=MMstat, method='REML') #method REML is
the most recommended
```

To show how the GAM looks using the `plot.gam( )` function (Fig. 9.31):

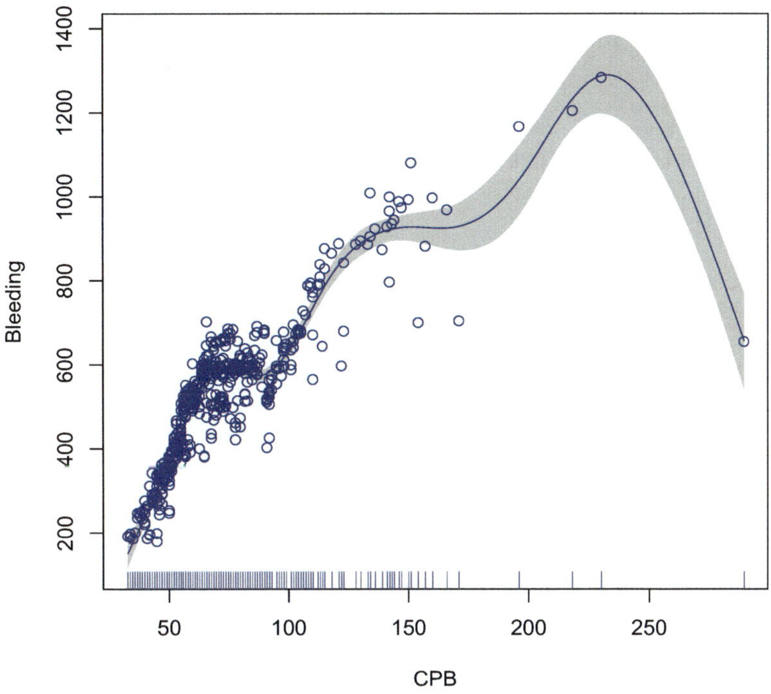

Fig. 9.31 Generalised additive model (GAM)

```
> plot.gam(modelgam, ylab='Bleeding',rug=TRUE, residuals = TRUE,
pch=1, cex=1, shade=TRUE, col='blue', shift=(coef(modelgam)[1]))
```

As you can see in Fig. 9.31, the curve now has some wiggles. Figure 9.32 summarises the output of the model:

```
> summary(modelgam)
```

The *a* in *gam* stands for *additive* which means no interactions. By definition we are not considering interaction effect at this level. Nevertheless, it is possible to include a factor for smoothing interaction using the `s(CPB, by=Aspirin)` function (one smooth for each category) or the `s(CPB, Age)` function for continuous variables.

Our model returned four variables as significant (`Broccoli`, `Aspirin`, `CPB` and `Age`). Do note that the explanatory `Broccoli` and `Age` variables are now statistically significant.

But how should I interpret the coefficients?

The first part of the output is not dissimilar to the one discussed before for the linear terms, where the results for the non-numeric explanatory variables are given with a coefficient and standard error. The second non-parametric part of the model is less intuitive to interpret. For this smoothing part, coefficients are not printed; this

```
Family: gaussian
Link function: identity

Formula:
Bleeding ~ Broccoli + s(CPB) + s(Age) + Male + Diabetes + Aspirin +
    s(Creatinine) + COPD + s(LVEF) + s(bmi)

Parametric coefficients:
            Estimate Std. Error t value Pr(>|t|)
(Intercept) 533.1736     5.8888  90.540  < 2e-16 ***
Broccoliy   -18.7163     5.6089  -3.337 0.000915 ***
Male1        -0.3393     5.2317  -0.065 0.948320
Diabetes1     4.2652     7.4396   0.573 0.566715
Diabetes2     0.6848    14.6469   0.047 0.962728
Aspirin1     22.9977     5.6921   4.040 6.24e-05 ***
COPD1       -19.7076    10.9640  -1.797 0.072902 .
---
Signif. codes:  0 '***' 0.001 '**' 0.01 '*' 0.05 '.' 0.1 ' ' 1

Approximate significance of smooth terms:
                edf Ref.df       F p-value
s(CPB)        8.597  8.943 363.587  <2e-16 ***
s(Age)        1.001  1.002   5.157  0.0235 *
s(Creatinine) 1.002  1.004   2.283  0.1310
s(LVEF)       1.002  1.004   2.956  0.0860 .
s(bmi)        1.002  1.003   2.638  0.1051
---
Signif. codes:  0 '***' 0.001 '**' 0.01 '*' 0.05 '.' 0.1 ' ' 1

R-sq.(adj) =   0.89   Deviance explained = 89.4%
-REML =   2651  Scale est. = 3213.7    n = 489
```

Fig. 9.32 Generalised additive model (GAM) summary

is because each smooth has several coefficients. Instead, effective degree of freedom (edf) is given. In essence, edf represents the complexity of the smooth (the higher the edf, the more complex), whereas an edf of 1 equals a straight line and 2 equals a quadratic curve.

We can perform more elegant plots as set out in Fig. 9.33 with the `plot_smooths( )` function:

```
> plot_smooths(modelgam=model,series=CPB, facet_terms=Aspirin,com
parison=Broccoli)
+theme(legend.position = "top")# library(tidymv)
```

This plot shows the smoothed relation between `CPB` time and `Bleeding` in the female vs male individuals grouped by `Aspirin` (1=yes). It is noteworthy that

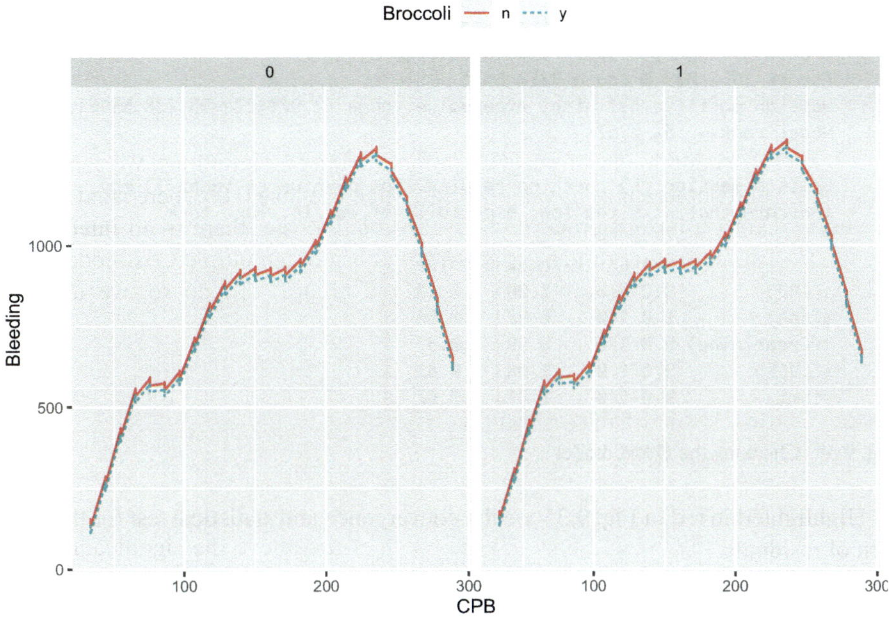

Fig. 9.33 Generalised additive model grouped by "Broccoli"

```
R-sq.(adj) =   0.89   Deviance explained = 89.4%
-REML =   2651  Scale est. = 3213.7     n = 489
```

Fig. 9.34 Generalised additive model and R-squared

bleeding non-linearly increases until a certain `CPB` time, then it decreases abruptly (perhaps because of the presence of outliers). The effect is not influenced by gender.

Now that the model is in place, we should check its validity before drawing final conclusions. The number of basis functions (k) determines how wiggly the model is. If there are not enough k basis functions, the curve might not capture enough data in the model. This results in suboptimal smoothing. Sometimes, visual inspection cannot provide a reliable answer; hence, we need to numerically test the model. *K* can be specified in the `s(..., k=..)` model. Or rather, `gam` function returns the optimal smoothing for us. The `gam` function also defaults to reporting the adjusted R-squared in the summary (Fig. 9.34):

Notably the model performance is good, considering the R-squared is equal to 0.89 (the model explains 89% of variability). However, we should carry out an in-depth analysis of the model performance with the `gam.check( )` function (Fig. 9.35):

```
> gam.check(modelgam)
```

How should we interpret the checked result?

```
Method: REML   Optimizer: outer newton
full convergence after 7 iterations.
Gradient range [-0.0005972456,0.001830878]
(score 2651.001 & scale 3213.655).
Hessian positive definite, eigenvalue range [2.973127e-05,238.5596].
Model rank =  52 / 52

Basis dimension (k) checking results. Low p-value (k-index<1) may
indicate that k is too low, especially if edf is close to k'.

                k' edf k-index p-value
s(CPB)         9.0 8.6    1.00    0.43
s(Age)         9.0 1.0    0.92    0.06 .
s(Creatinine) 9.0 1.0    0.99    0.37
s(LVEF)        9.0 1.0    1.03    0.81
s(bmi)         9.0 1.0    1.01    0.62
```

Fig. 9.35 Checking the GAM model

Highlighted in red in Fig. 9.35 are the convergence and statistical test for the pattern of residuals.

- *Full convergence:* "R" has found the best solution (too many parameters for not enough data may undermine the convergence).
- *Statistical test for the pattern of residuals:* a small p-value may indicate that there are not enough basis functions (k) and therefore [no/little] presence of pattern in the residuals.

Notably, the number of k for the `Age` variable is on the low side, yet the p-value is 0.06.

Visual inspection of the residuals is also important, and the same `gam.check()` function returns four plots:

1. *Plot for model residuals:* a QQ plot which compares model residuals to normal distribution (see Fig. 9.36).
2. *Histogram of GAM residuals:* with residuals that should be fairly normal (see Fig. 9.37).
3. *Scatterplot of GAM residuals:* whereby residual values should be evenly distributed around zero (see Fig. 9.38).
4. *Response vs fitted value:* a perfect model would form a straight line and we would expect the pattern to cluster around a 1 to 1 line (see Fig. 9.39).

Lastly, we may want to check for concurvity that is the non-parametric analogue of multicollinearity. "Concurvity occurs when some smooth term in a model could be approximated by one or more of the other smooth terms in the model".

Concurvity measure spans from 0, suggesting no problem, to 1, indicating that the function lies entirely in the space of one or more of the other smooth terms (Fig. 9.40).

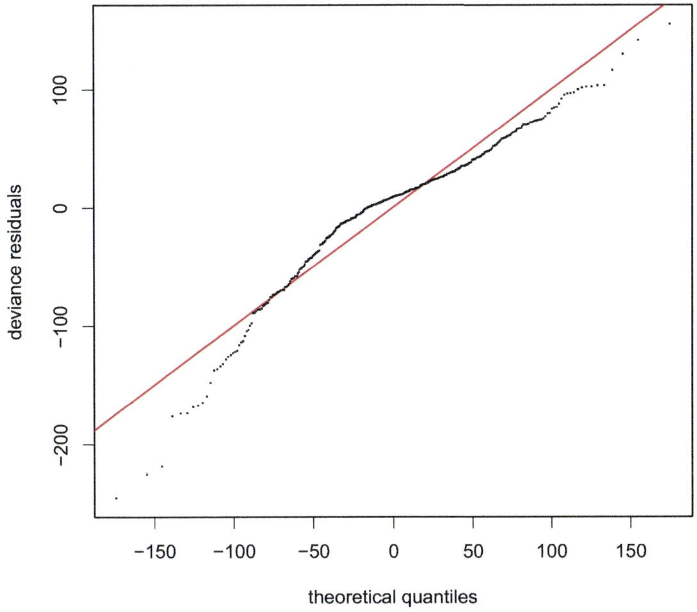

Fig. 9.36 Quantile-quantile plot that compares model GAM residuals to normal distribution

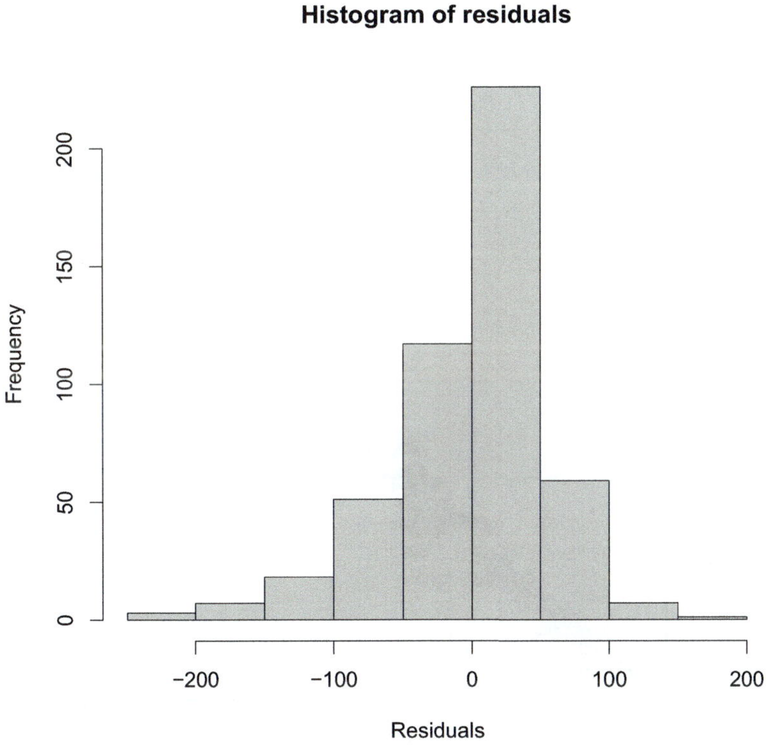

Fig. 9.37 Histogram of GAM residuals

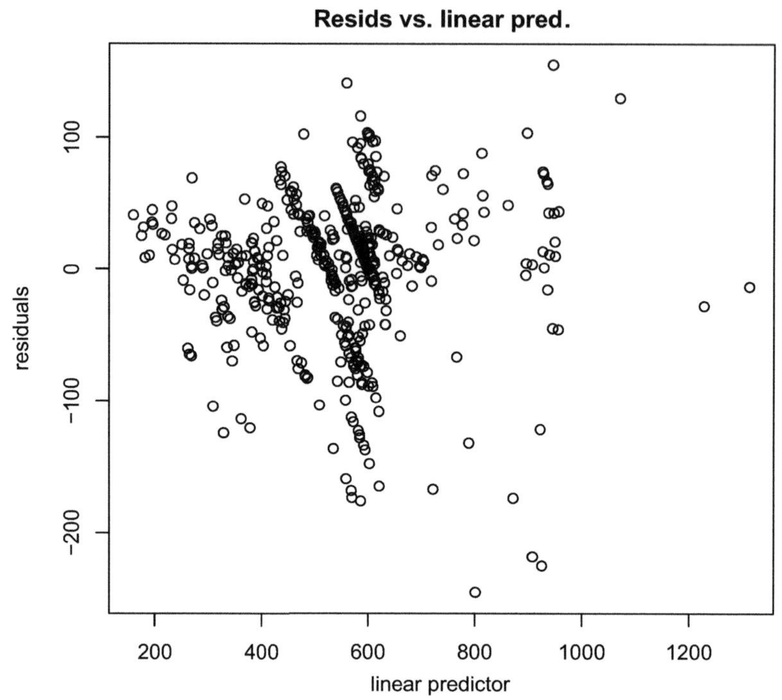

Fig. 9.38 Scatterplot of GAM residuals

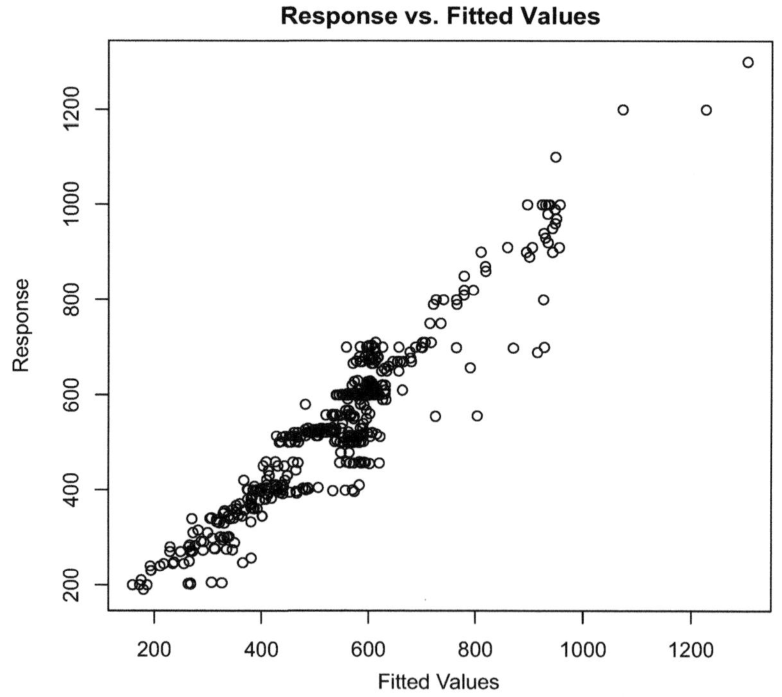

Fig. 9.39 Response vs fitted values

```
              para     s(CPB)    s(Age) s(Creatinine)    s(LVEF)     s(bmi)
worst    0.8230496 0.2532547 0.2169974      0.2034238 0.1917182 0.1510579
observed 0.8230496 0.2104918 0.1743549      0.1868080 0.0979581 0.1155071
estimate 0.8230496 0.1749562 0.1575430      0.1529703 0.1039801 0.1007373
```

Fig. 9.40 Concurvity analysis

We should always check the first line (*worst*), for no explanatory variables are affected by concurvity.

We conclude that `CPB`, `Aspirin`, `Broccoli` and `Age` are the variables that influence the post-operative `Bleeding`, according to the GAM model we have built.

9.20 Data Mining with Stepwise Model Selection

At this stage I go back a little, facing again the problem of what variables to include in the model. We have previously stated that we include the explanatory *variables of interest*, with no statistical pre-screening. This is probably the most logical way to proceed. If a predictor is known from literature, and previous research, to influence our dependent variable, then it must be included in our model—regardless of the level of statistical significance at bivariate pre-screening.

However, we may face problems when the dataset has many variables. There are some techniques that apply automatically.

Stepwise regression (also known as *stepwise selection*) is an iterative process that *adds* and *removes* predictors in the predictive model. It does so to find the subset of variables in the dataset which make up the optimal performing model.

There are three strategies to stepwise regression:

1. *Forward selection* `direction = 'forward'`*:* the starting point is *no predictors*. Then the process consists of adding the most influential predictors until the improvement is no longer statistically significant.
2. *Backward selection or elimination* `direction = 'backward'`*:* the starting point is the *full model*. Then the least influential predictors are eliminated until all predictors are statistically significant.
3. *Sequential replacement or stepwise regression* `direction = 'both'`*:* is a combination of the two above. It starts like the forward model with no predictors and the most influential variables are added. After adding each of the new variables, the process removes any variables that provide any improvement in the model (similarly to the backward selection).

Backward elimination is the least *offensive*; hence, it is the one which I cover here.

There are a few packages in "R" for this purpose. Below I use the `step( )` function provided in the built-in package in "R". This process is sensitive to missing values; hence, in order to proceed we should remove them with the `na.omit( )` function (Fig. 9.41).

```
> MMnomiss= na.omit(MMstat)# Omitting missing values
analysisfull<-lm(Bleeding~Broccoli+CPB+Age+Male+Diabetes+Aspirin+
Creatinine+COPD+LVEF
+bmi,data=MMnomiss)#creating the new model from MMnomiss
> newabackward<-step(analysisfull, trace=FALSE, direction =
'backward')
> summary(newabackward)
```

By selecting the `trace=TRUE` option, "R" returns the entire selection steps from the model which go from the highest AIC to the lowest (not shown in this section). In this case it spans from 1644.2 to 1633.5.

Below I report only the starting point (full model) and the final model with the lowest AIC (Fig. 9.42).

```
Call:
lm(formula = Bleeding ~ Broccoli + CPB + Aspirin, data = MMnomiss)

Residuals:
    Min      1Q  Median      3Q     Max
-744.24  -49.72    9.60   68.51  231.67

Coefficients:
            Estimate Std. Error t value Pr(>|t|)
(Intercept)  203.889     25.019   8.149 7.25e-14 ***
Broccoliy    -30.609     16.818  -1.820  0.07049 .
CPB            4.212      0.270  15.601  < 2e-16 ***
Aspirin1      47.644     15.849   3.006  0.00304 **
---
Signif. codes:  0 '***' 0.001 '**' 0.01 '*' 0.05 '.' 0.1 ' ' 1

Residual standard error: 102.5 on 172 degrees of freedom
Multiple R-squared:  0.6541,	Adjusted R-squared:  0.6481
F-statistic: 108.4 on 3 and 172 DF,  p-value: < 2.2e-16
```

Fig. 9.41 Stepwise linear regression

```
Start:  AIC=1644.23
Bleeding ~ Broccoli + CPB + Age + Male + Diabetes + Aspirin +
    Creatinine + COPD + LVEF + bmi


Step:  AIC=1633.57
Bleeding ~ Broccoli + CPB + Aspirin
```

Fig. 9.42 Final AIC value

In stepwise selection, the privilege of selecting the variables to be included in the full model is best left to the *machine algorithm* (data mining). Specifically, we should aim to include the predictors of interest, according to our knowledge.

9.21 Conclusions

"All models are wrong, some of them are useful". This is a very famous statement. Linear regression allows you to build a model where the *dependent variable* is *numeric* and yet the explanatory variables can be a combination of numeric and non-numeric. We often use linear regression in medicine, since many outcomes of interest are numeric such as length of in hospital stay, amount of bleeding, etc. Linear regression output returns beta coefficients. These coefficients tell us how much the dependent variable varies, as the independent variable increases by 1 unit, while keeping all other variables constant.

However, there are some assumptions to validate, and before interpreting the results we should analyse the residuals. Importantly, residuals should be normally distributed (homoscedasticity). If not, we may try to transform the dependent variables or the independent variables. A few types of data transformation may apply, such as log or polynomial, Box-Cox transformation or even removing any influential observations.

You are also introduced to the generalised additive model (GAM), which can combine both linear and non-linear terms.

Further Readings

Ciaburro G. Regression analysis with R: design and develop statistical nodes to identify unique relationships within data at scale. Birmingham: Packt Publishing; 2018.

Faraway JJ. Linear models with R. Boca Raton, FL: CRC Press; 2016.

Hoffmann JP. Linear regression models: applications in R. Boca Raton, FL: CRC Press; 2021.

Kim AY, Ismay C. Statistical inference via data science: a modern dive into R and the tidyverse. Boca Raton, FL: CRC Press; 2019.

Lilja D. Linear regression using R: an introduction to data modeling. Minneapolis, MN: University of Minnesota Libraries Publishing [Imprint]; 2016.

Sengupta D, Jammalamadaka SR. Linear models and regression with R: an integrated approach. Singapore: World Scientific Publishing Company; 2019.

Sheather S, Verwoerd CDA, Oostrom CG. A modern approach to regression with R. New York: Springer; 1979.

Wood SN. Fast stable restricted maximum likelihood and marginal likelihood estimation of semiparametric generalized linear models. J R Stat Soc B. 2011;73(1):3–36.

Chapter 10
Logistic Regression

Logistic Regression

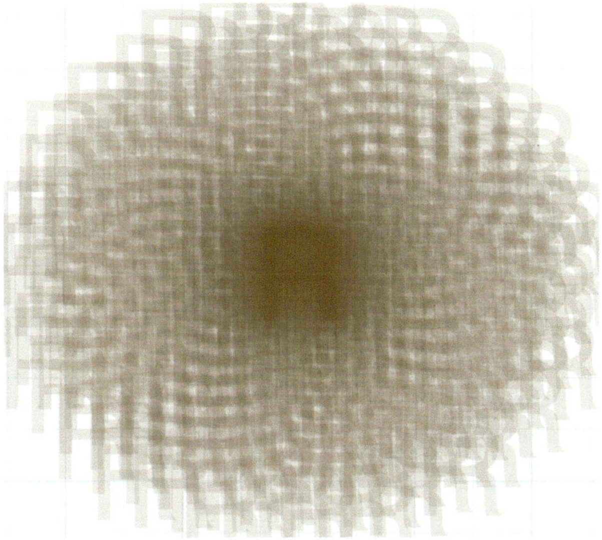

10.1 Software and R-Packages Required for This Chapter

If you haven't already, you need to download and install base-R and R-studio as set out in Chap. 2 under the heading "Downloading "R" and R-studio".

The relevant R-packages needed for this chapter are:

- tidyverse—it can be downloaded at:
- http://tidyverse.tidyverse.org
- tableone—it can be downloaded at:

M. Moscarelli, *Biostatistics With 'R': A Guide for Medical Doctors*,
https://doi.org/10.1007/978-3-031-33073-5_10

- https://github.com/kaz-yos/tableone
- epiDisplay—it can be downloaded at:
- Repository: CRAN
- pscl—it can be downloaded at:
- http://github.com/atahk/pscl
- ROCR—it can be downloaded at:
- http://ipa-tys.github.io/ROCR
- pROC—it can be downloaded at:
- http://expasy.org/tools/pROC
- ResourceSelection—it can be downloaded at:
- https://github.com/psolymos/ResourceSelection
- sjPlot—it can be downloaded at:
- https://strengejacke.github.io/sjPlot
- gridExtra—it can be downloaded at:
- Repository: CRAN

10.2 Where to Download the Example Dataset and Script for This Chapter

If you haven't already downloaded the supplementary dataset named `MMstat.csv` created as a practical example for use throughout this book, you will find it at the link that follows. The script for this chapter named `Chapter 10. Logistic regression.R` can also be found and downloaded at the following link:

https://github.com/mmlondon77/Biobook.git.

10.3 Logistic Regression

Logistic regression is also known as *binary logistic regression*, *binomial logistic regression* or *logit model* and is used when the outcome of interest is *binary*.

This is a very common scenario in medicine. As doctors, we are very often interested in modelling outcomes such as death (dead/alive) and whether patients had specific post-operative complications (y/n) or cancer relapse after surgery (y/n). Those are all binary outcomes.

On the contrary, linear regression is used when the outcome of interest is numeric (e.g. amount of post-operative bleeding, days spent in the intensive care unit, etc.). Linear regression was covered in Chap. 9. However, I set out here the differences between the two techniques and why linearity methods should not be applied to logistic regression.

You can see from Fig. 10.1, in the plot for logistic regression (the plot on the left), the dependent variable/outcome of interest is binary, it is the `Mortality` variable from our `MMstat` dataset, and it is coded as 1 = dead and 0 = alive and is shown on the y-axis. The explanatory variable is of a continuous nature; it is the `CC` variable (cross-clamp/ischaemic time) from the example dataset and is shown on the x-axis. If we run this linear regression model with the binary `Mortality` variable and the continuous explanatory `CC` variable, the model plots a straight line through these points. As you can see, this model does not fit the data at all, since the line is somewhere between the points located at 0 and 1, therefore returning impossible predicted values between 0 and 1.

However, for linear regression (Fig. 10.1, on the right) the dependent variable/outcome of interest is numeric; it is the `Bleeding` variable from the example dataset and is shown on the y-axis. The independent/explanatory variable is also numeric; it is the `CC` variable from the example dataset and is shown on the x-axis. The red line (line of best fit) created by minimising the differences between the observations (with least squares method) attempts to describe the predicted values. The model is not optimal, since many values of the dependent `CC` variable lie far from the line, but it is a reasonable attempt.

For a binary outcome, we are interested in modelling the proportion of patients with the outcome of interest (proportion of patients who died in hospital after surgery), i.e. the probability of a patient dying after surgery.

However, probabilities are continuous numbers and they can only take values from 0 to 1. In this case, a linear model for a binary outcome would predict an erroneous number, in some cases above 1 or below 0.

We need a statistical trick to convert the variable of interest into one that can be modelled in a regression equation. We do so thanks to the *link function*. The most used link function is the *logit*. In simple words, rather than *directly* modelling the probability, we in fact model the *logit* of the probability. The formula used is:

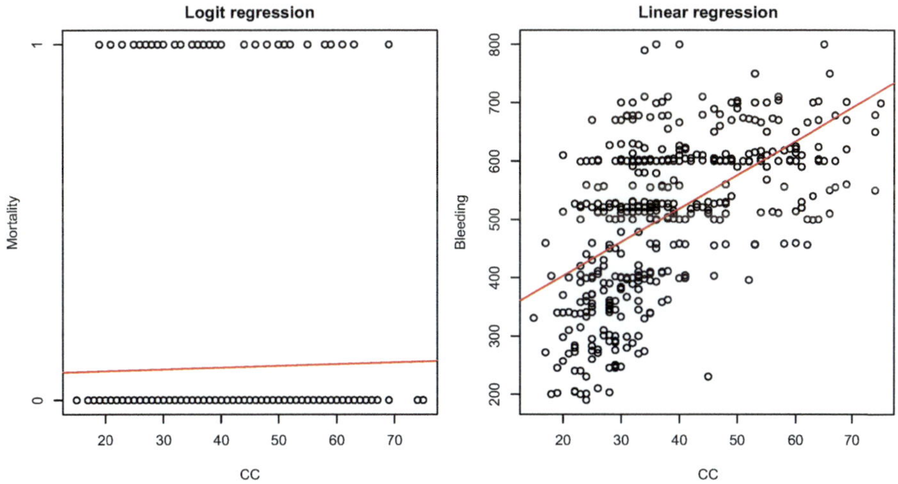

Fig. 10.1 A depiction of the clear difference between logit regression (left) and linear regression (right)

$$\text{logit}(p) = \log\left(\frac{p}{1-p}\right) = \log(\text{odds})$$

If we convert the y-axis to log we can run a regression model in a similar way to linear regression. Still the predicted values for probabilities are given between 0 and 1 after exponentiating them (antilog).

In simple words, logistic regression values on the y-axis are confined to 0 (absence of outcome) or 1 (presence of outcome). We are interested in the probability of a certain event happening, given a certain explanatory variable. To do so, we transform the y-axis to be log odds instead of probability (Fig. 10.2), with the function logit = $\log(p/(1-p))$.

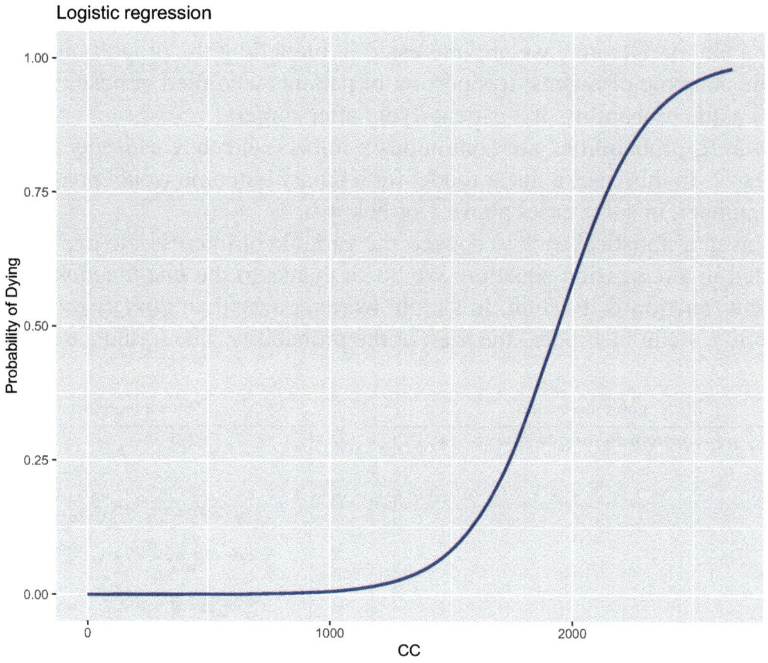

Fig. 10.2 Logit regression—the link function allows us to model the dependent variable as log(odds), while the sigmoid function maps any predicted values of probabilities into another value between 0 and 1

10.4 Odds and Probability

Logistic regression models *odds*, instead of *probability*.

Log odds can take any values (negative and positive), while probability spans only from 0 to 1. We need log odds (rather than simple odds) to do the calculus. After calculus, the log(odds) can be exponentiated (antilog), transformed to odds and finally interpreted.

Let me explain the difference between odds and probability with the aid of the table that follows:

In the example provided in Table 10.1, we have 32 patients assigned to the broccoli treatment. Those are the patients who commenced a strict broccoli dietary regimen 1 week prior to cardiac surgery. Amongst this broccoli group, one individual bled significantly after surgery. For the control group (no broccoli/liberal dietary regimen), amongst 28 patients 7 individuals bled significantly after surgery, while 21 did not.

The probability or *absolute risk* of an event is the likelihood of an occurrence of that event in the population of risk. The absolute risk of bleeding in the broccoli population is 1/32 = *A/n1* (1 patient out of 32 bled) = 0.03 or 3%. The absolute risk of bleeding in the no-broccoli population is 7/28 = *C/n2* (7 patients out of 28 bled) = 0.25 or 25%.

The odds of bleeding in the experimental group (broccoli group) are 1/31 = 0.03 (note that the denominator is not the total amount of individuals in the broccoli group, rather the number of patients who did not bleed = *A/B*). The odds of bleeding in the control group are 7/21 = 0.33 = *C/D*.

The odds ratio (OR) is intuitively calculated as below:

$$\text{Odds Ratio} = \frac{A/B\left(\text{odds of broccoli}\right)}{C/D\left(\text{odds of no broccoli}\right)} = \frac{AD}{BD}$$

Therefore, in this case, the OR is 0.03/0.33=0.09. Specifically, the odds of bleeding for patients who had broccoli are 0.09 to 1. How to express an OR of 0.09? Had this been considered risk, we could say that broccoli reduces the risk of bleeding by 91%.

However, because it is expressed as OR, we must say that for every 0.09 person who bled in the broccoli group, 1 person bled in the no-broccoli group (in other words, for every 9 people who include the broccoli dietary regimen prior to surgery,

Table 10.1

	Bleeding after surgery	No bleeding after surgery	Total
Had broccoli before surgery	1 (A)	31 (B)	32 (n1)
No broccoli before surgery	7 (C)	21 (D)	28 (n2)
Total	8	52	60

and who bleed significantly after surgery, 100 people consuming a liberal diet will probably bleed). Thus, the odds are 9 to 100 (or 0.09 to 1).

10.5 Cross-Tabulation

Before we assemble the logit model and start delving into it, we should once again explore in-depth our `MMstat` dataset and understand how each explanatory variable relates to the dependent variable. By cross-tabulating, I demonstrate the process of exploring the relationships between the dependent variable (in our case `Mortality`) to all other explanatory variables/covariates in the dataset. Such covariates can be numeric or non-numeric. The latter can be expressed as proportion in relation to the binary outcome (e.g. percentage of male and female who died), whereas the numeric covariates can be summarised as mean or median if the sample is normally or not-normally distributed, respectively (e.g. mean age of patients who died and survived/median cardio-pulmonary bypass). This process is part of explanatory data analysis, and as I explained in its dedicated chapter, we can use the `CreateTableOne( )` function from the `tableone` package (Fig. 10.3):

```
                         Stratified by Mortality
                          0                          1                          p      test
  n                          456                         44
  Age (median [IQR])       66.00 [55.75, 73.00]   59.50 [51.00, 66.00]   0.001 nonnorm
  Weight (mean (SD))       74.30 (14.03)          75.89 (12.40)          0.469
  Height (mean (SD))      167.20 (9.14)          169.89 (10.03)          0.065
  LVEF (median [IQR])      55.00 [50.00, 56.00]   55.00 [48.75, 60.00]   0.785 nonnorm
  Creatinine (mean (SD))   0.89 (0.30)             0.82 (0.19)           0.128
  CPB (median [IQR])       67.00 [54.00, 84.00]   70.00 [56.50, 78.25]   0.967 nonnorm
  CC (median [IQR])        20.00 [14.00, 34.00]   22.50 [13.00, 33.50]   0.916 nonnorm
  Bleeding (mean (SD))    539.67 (174.17)        526.73 (154.60)         0.635
  Broccoli = y (%)           198 (43.4)              5 (11.4)           <0.001
  Male = 1 (%)               200 (43.9)             24 (54.5)            0.229
  Diabetes (%)                                                           0.325
     0                       377 (82.7)             36 (81.8)
     1                        66 (14.5)              5 (11.4)
     2                        13 ( 2.9)              3 ( 6.8)
  Aspirin = 1 (%)            300 (65.8)             29 (65.9)            1.000
  LOS (median [IQR])       11.00 [7.00, 21.00]    15.00 [7.50, 21.00]    0.558 nonnorm
  COPD (%)                                                               0.534
     0                       418 (91.7)             42 (95.5)
     1                        27 ( 5.9)              2 ( 4.5)
     NA                       11 ( 2.4)              0 ( 0.0)
```

Fig. 10.3 Cross-tabulation using tableone, to visualise the relationship between numeric and non-numeric variables and the binary mortality outcome

```
> varsToFactor <- c("Male","Diabetes","Mortality","Aspirin",
"COPD")# convert variable to factors
```

```
> MMstat[varsToFactor] <- lapply(MMstat[varsToFactor], factor)#
use the function lapply to pass the converted variable to the data-
set MMstat
> vars<- c('Age', 'Weight', 'Height', 'LVEF', 'Creatinine', 'CPB',
'CC', 'Bleeding', 'Broccoli', "Male","Diabetes","Aspirin", 'LOS',
'COPD')#creating the object 'vars'
> tableOne <- CreateTableOne(vars = vars, strata = c("Mortality"),
data = MMstat, includeNA = TRUE)# creating the object tableOne with
the function CreateTableOne
> tableOne
> summary(tableOne)
> Nonnormal<-c('Age', 'CPB', 'CC', 'LVEF', 'LOS')# specifying the
non-normal variables
> print(tableOne, nonnormal=Nonnormal)#printing the final table
```

As we can tell from Fig. 10.3, the vast majority of proportion and indices of central tendency (mean and median) do not significantly differ between individuals who died ($n = 44$) and those who survived ($n = 456$). Interestingly, individuals who died were of a younger age. This initial cross-tabulation is of interest since it already highlights a difference in mortality, when considering the proportions in the broccoli vs no-broccoli groups. Only a few patients who included `Broccoli` before surgery died (11.4%). No other differences (e.g. gender differences) were noticed. Notably, the `tableone` function also returns the associated p-value.

10.6 Simple Logistic Regression

Simple logistic regression is a model based on a single predictor. It is sometimes used to explore time trend, for instance, modelling the mortality rate in relation to years of surgery. In this case the question would be: does mortality rate increase over the years?

Since logistic regression belongs to the generalised linear model (GLM), the "R" `glm( )` function is used, and we must specify a few parameters:

- Dependent variable: must be binary.
- Predictor/explanatory variable: can be either numeric or non-numeric and is coded after the tilde ~.
- Distribution: binomial; the command is `family='binomial'`.
- Link function: to transform the dependent variable, the most used is *logit*; the command is `link='logit'`.

Importantly, for continuous variables, we do not assume that they have to follow a normal distribution. However, the relationship between the explanatory variable and the response variable *has to be linear*. Let us say we want to model the relationship between `Mortality` and `Age`. We then assume that the mortality rate changes by the same amount for every unit increase in `Age` (years) and no curve is allowed (a linear relationship).

Below is an example of simple logistic regression, modelling the dependent `Mortality` variable against the independent `Age` variable:

```
> str(MMstat$Mortality)#checking the structure of the outcome of
interest
> simplemodel<-glm(Mortality~Age, family = 'binomial'(link=logit),
data=MMstat)
```

Before interpreting the results using `summary(simplemodel)`, we should perform more cross-tabulation. By exploring the relationship between the categorical `Mortality` variable and the explanatory continuous `Age` variable, we can find out whether or not a linear relationship exists. Since `Mortality` is categorical, we should calculate the odds of `Mortality` by `Age` with a *frequency table*, transform it to log(odds) and plot it against the `Age` variable as shown in the plot below (Fig. 10.4):

By observing the plot, we might hypothesise an inverse linear relationship (with no *curves*) between `Mortality` and `Age` (i.e. post-operative `Mortality` decreases as `Age` increases). In fact, if we go back to Fig. 10.3, the median age of individuals who died was lower than the median of individuals who survived. Now we can go ahead and run the `summary` command (Fig. 10.5):

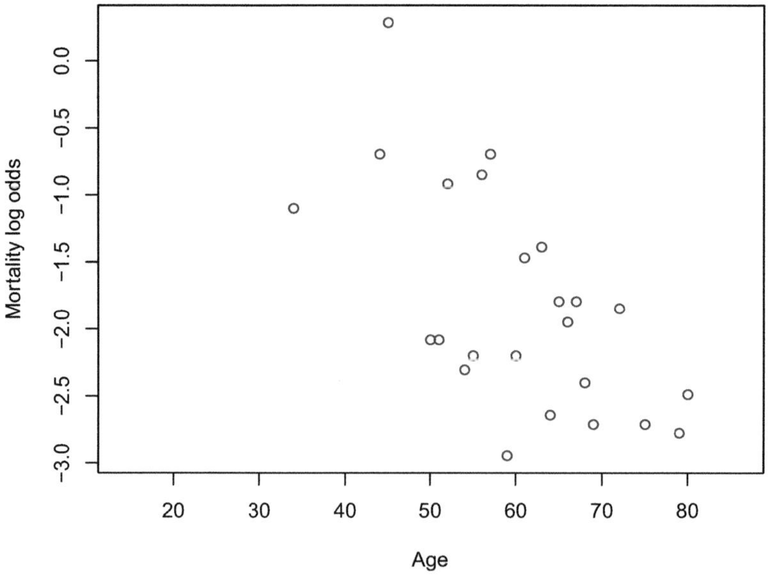

Fig. 10.4 Checking the linearity assumption between the dependent Mortality variable and the independent Age variable, with Mortality reported in log(odds)

```
> summary(simplemodel)
```

The `summary` function returns the estimate of the intercept and the numeric `Age` variable as log(odds). We interpret the estimate/coefficient for `Age`, as the increase/decrease in log(odds) of the risk of dying, for every 1-year increase in `Age`.

Logistic regression output is however reported in odds ratio (OR). If we exponentiate the coefficient, we obtain the OR as below:

```
> round(exp(-0.02), digits = 2)# exponentiate or anti log of the
estimate to obtain the OR
[1] 0.98# odds ratio for Age
```

This is also statistically significant since the associated p-value is p=0.007.

Let us perform a logistic regression, this time with a categorical variable such as `Broccoli` (Fig. 10.6):

```
>        simplemodel2<-glm(Mortality~Broccoli,        family        =
'binomial'(link=logit), data=MMstat)
> summary(simplemodel2)
```

The summary gives the log(odds) associated to `Broccoliy` (the individuals who consumed `Broccoli` before cardiac surgery), and if we exponentiate the estimate we obtain the OR:

```
> round(exp(-1.78), digits = 2)
[1] 0.17# OR of the Broccoli group.
```

```
Coefficients:
             Estimate Std. Error z value Pr(>|z|)
(Intercept) -0.51181    0.67589  -0.757  0.44890
Age         -0.02991    0.01116  -2.680  0.00737 **
---
Signif. codes:  0 '***' 0.001 '**' 0.01 '*' 0.05 '.' 0.1 ' ' 1
```

Fig. 10.5 Summary of simple logistic model with Mortality as dependent variable and Age as continuous explanatory variable

```
Coefficients:
             Estimate Std. Error z value Pr(>|z|)
(Intercept)  -1.8894     0.1718 -10.997  < 2e-16 ***
Broccoliy    -1.7894     0.4843  -3.695  0.00022 ***
---
Signif. codes:  0 '***' 0.001 '**' 0.01 '*' 0.05 '.' 0.1 ' ' 1
```

Fig. 10.6 Summary of simple logistic model with Mortality as the dependent variable and Age as the continuous explanatory variable

```
Logistic regression predicting Mortality : 1 vs 0

                   OR(95%CI)          P(Wald's test) P(LR-test)
Age (cont. var.) 0.97 (0.95,0.99)  0.007          0.009

Log-likelihood = -145.5063
No. of observations = 500
AIC value = 295.0126
```

Fig. 10.7 Logistic.display function returns OR along with 95% confidence interval

The odds for mortality for the `Broccoli` group are 0.17 the odds for the control (no-Broccoli). Do also note that this is highly significant since the p-value is tiny (=0.00022).

The `epiDisplay` package allows a fast and easy conversion to OR (Fig. 10.7):

```
> logistic.display(simplemodel, alpha = 0.05, crude = FALSE,
crude.p.value = FALSE, decimal = 2, simplified = FALSE)
```

The `logistic.display` function returns the OR along with 95% CI and p-value.

10.7 Logistic Regression Assumptions

Before moving towards the stage of including multiple predictors, let me clarify the assumptions that must hold in the context of logistic regression. Those are:

(a) Linearity between the numeric predictors and the dependent variable given in log(odds)
(b) Absence of multicollinearity
(c) Lack of strongly influential outliers
(d) Independency of observations

With regard to *linearity*, we have already plotted the `Age` variable against the log(odds) of `Mortality`. Let us try to plot all the numerical variables at once to check for linearity (the code is provided in the script for this chapter) (Fig. 10.8).

Many explanatory variables show a non-linear relationship with the `Mortality` log(odds). As an example, let us scrutinise the relationship between `Bleeding` and `Mortality`. Intuitively it is not linear and may need some transformation. The Box-Tidwell test is used to test linearity between the continuous variable and the log odds of the dependent variable; however, this is beyond the scope of this book.

In Chap. 9 on linear regression, I explained how to transform variables to obtain linearity (log, cubic, Box-Cox transformation). However, considering the scarcity of events, it only included the `Age` variable.

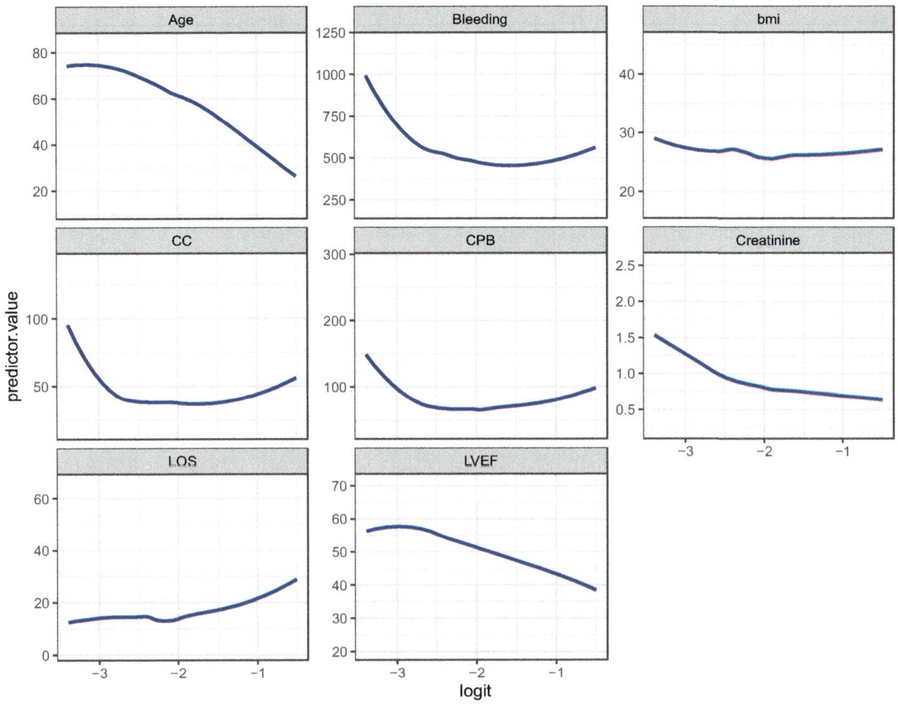

Fig. 10.8 Exploration of linearity—correlation between independent variables and log(odds) of the dependent Mortality variable

Multicollinearity is also covered in Chap. 9. This is the case when variables are highly correlated and the variance can't be partitioned between them. Later in this chapter I will again explain how to check for multicollinearity for our chosen *multivariable logistic regression model.*

Not all *unusual points* affect a regression model. As was discussed in linear regression in Chap. 9, a data point has high *leverage* when it has extreme predictor *x* values (more extreme compared to the rest of the observations). In fact, an *outlier* is a data point whose response *y* value does not follow the general trend of the rest of the data. Such data points are *influential* if they affect or influence any part of regression analysis.

If we have a look at Fig. 10.9, we might be able to understand the differences between *outliers* and *high leverage data points*. Outliers do not follow the bulk of the other data points; they stand out on the y-axis (with high residuals) (see Fig. 10.9a). A data point with high leverage can follow the trend, but represent extreme values on the x-axis (see Fig. 10.9b). When a data point has an extreme x-value and also high residual (on the y-axis), it can significantly modify the regression line; hence, it is coded as an *influential point* (see Fig. 10.9c).

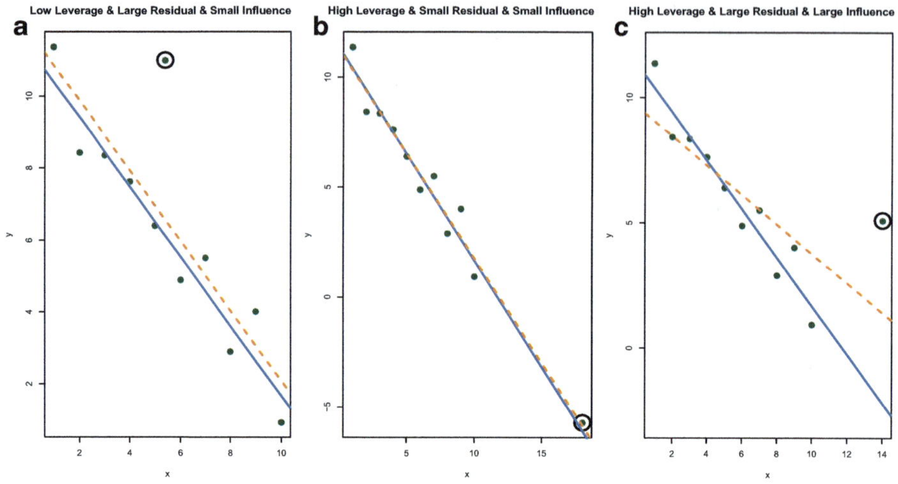

Fig. 10.9 (**a**) *Outlier*, a data point with large residual (far from the line of best fit); (**b**) *high leverage* data point, extreme observation on the x-axis, yet showing the same direction of the other observations since it lies close to the line of best fit; (**c**) *influential observation* with both large residual and high leverage. The blue line represents the regression line of the original data. In all three plots, the dotted lines represent the regression line after we add the unusual observation. Note that only in Fig. 10.9c the line of best fit significantly changes

Cook's distance is an estimate of the influence of a data point. The measurement is a combination of each observation's leverage and residual values; the higher the leverage and residuals, the higher the Cook's distance.

Standardised residual is used to determine whether a data point is an outlier or not. Data points with absolute standardised residual values greater than 3 may represent possible significant outliers.

The Cook's distance is considered high if it is greater than 0.5 and extreme if it is greater than 1. Another more conservative approach is to explore all the data points with a Cook's distance above 4/n, where n is the number of the observation in the dataset.

We should always plot the Cook's distance for the chosen model. Let us check the Cook's distance in the `simplemodel` we built:

```
>  simplemodel<-glm(Mortality~Age,family='binomial'(link=logit),
data=MMstat)
> plot(simplemodel, which = 4, id.n = 5)# showing the top 5 influ-
ential variables
```

Figure 10.10 depicts the five most influential data points (rows 132, 164, 329, 342, 428). They are all below 0.5; hence, with regard to the simple model, no *significant* influential points were detected.

We can now visualise them with the code below (Fig. 10.11):

```
> model.data <- augment(simplemodel) %>%
```

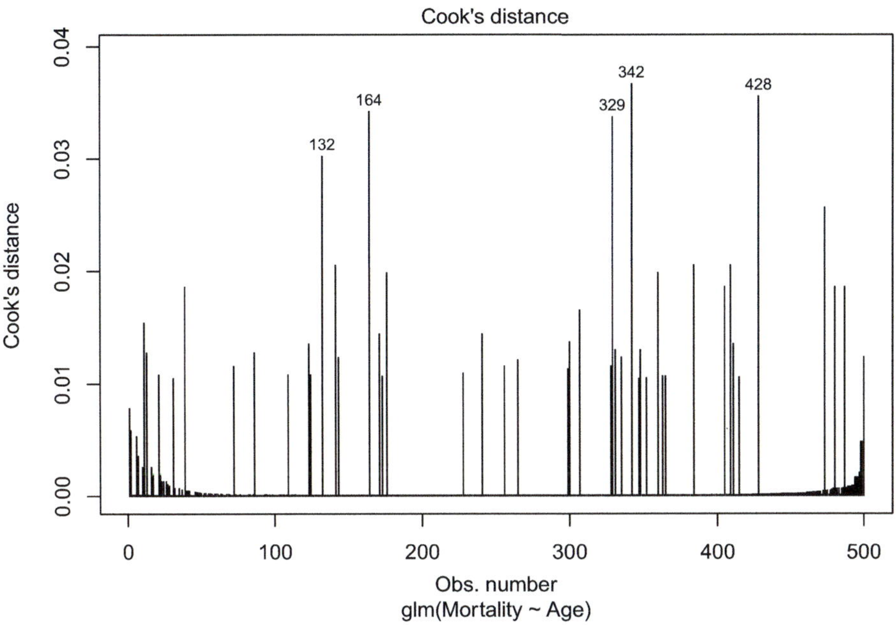

Fig. 10.10 Evaluating the presence of influential data points by calculating the Cook's distance

	Mortality	Age	.fitted	.resid	.std.resid	.hat	.sigma	.cooksd	index
	<fct>	<int>	<dbl>	<dbl>	<dbl>	<dbl>	<dbl>	<dbl>	<int>
1	1	37	-1.62	1.90	1.91	0.0117	0.760	0.0302	132
2	1	79	-2.87	2.42	2.43	0.00384	0.757	0.0343	164
3	1	35	-1.56	1.87	1.88	0.0138	0.761	0.0338	329
4	1	80	-2.90	2.43	2.44	0.00399	0.757	0.0367	342
5	1	34	-1.53	1.86	1.87	0.0150	0.761	0.0356	428

Fig. 10.11 Visualising the top 5 data points with the highest Cook's distance

```
  mutate(index = 1:n())
model.data %>% top_n(5, .cooksd)# visualizing the 5 values with
the highest Cooks'D.
```

Finally, *independence of errors* requires that there be no dependence between samples in the model, e.g. using the same individuals at different times, as in the case of repeated measures.

10.8 Multiple Logistic Regression

If we fit several explanatory variables at once, we obtain a multiple regression model. As per linear regression, explanatory variables can be both numeric and non-numeric.

But which and how many variables to include in the model? As a rule of thumb one predictive variable can be studied for every ten events. How many events in our dataset? Since the event of interest is `Mortality`, we can use the `table( )` function:

```
> table(MMstat$Mortality)
0   1
456  44
```

We have 44 events. In order to avoid overfitting, which would render the model unstable (not robust), we will include only four explanatory variables. Below is the script for `multimodel` multivariable logistic regression:

```
> multimodel<-glm(Mortality~Broccoli+Age+Male+Diabetes,family='bi
nomial'(link=logit), data=MMstat)
```

Since we want to continue with a logistic model, the only numeric variable we include is `Age`. For all others there is a certain degree of non-linearity between the log(dependent) and independent continuous variables. Based on our knowledge, gender, diabetes and obviously age may impact mortality, hence were included. The model includes the `Broccoli` covariate as part of the original research question.

10.9 Full Model Interpretation

With the `summary( )` function we can finally run the model and analyse the results (Fig 10.12):

```
> multimodel<-glm(Mortality~Broccoli+Age+Male+Diabetes,family='bi
nomial'(link=logit), data=MMstat)
> summary(multimodel)
```

- `Estimate`: outlines the regression coefficients. They are given in log(odds). They must be antilog (exponentiated) to return ORs.
- `Standard Error`: low standard errors are advisable. There is no general consensus on how low they must be, yet below 1 is recommended.
- `Z value`: sets out the standard deviations from the means, e.g. the z-value for `Broccoli` is 3.6 SD, which incidentally is well below the 95% confidence interval (1.96 SD), indicating statistical significance.
- `Pr(>|z|)`: represents the p-values of statistical significance.

The model also returns the deviance of the residuals. This is helpful for a quick check to understand the distribution of the residuals above and below the median.

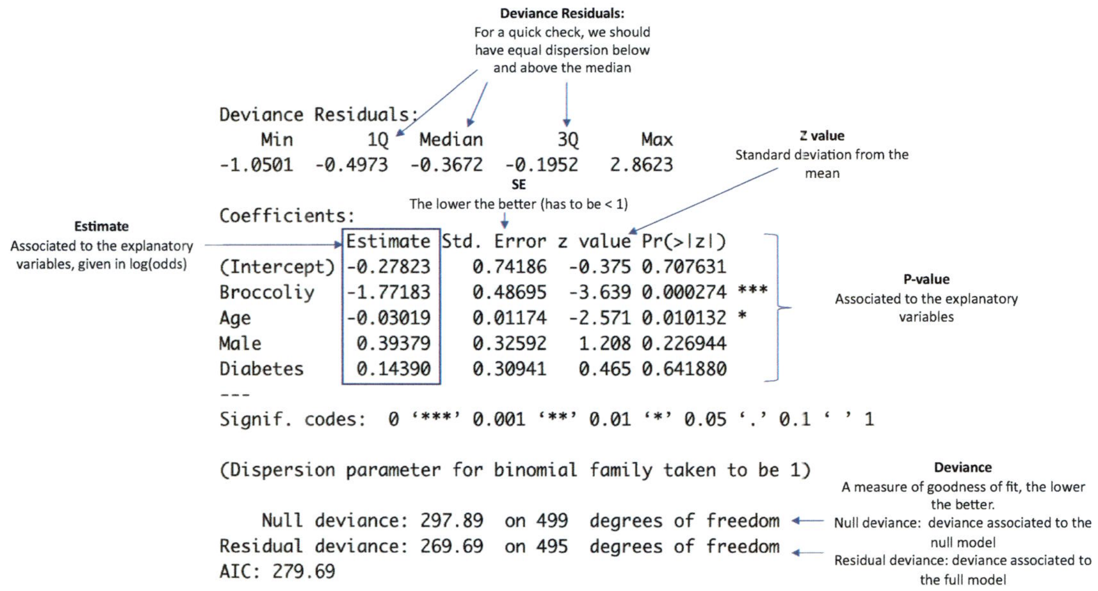

Fig. 10.12 Summary output of the multivariable logit regression

Finally, the deviance as a measure of goodness of fit is also given. We will cover *deviance* in a dedicated section later in this chapter.

How to exponentiate log(odds)? There are many functions. However, it is also helpful to plot both the *log* and *unlog* values of the coefficient as set out in Fig. 10.13:

```
> OR<-plot_model(multimodel, transform = 'exp', show.values =
TRUE)# from the package sjPlot.
> lOR<-plot_model(multimodel, transform = NULL, show.values = TRUE)
> grid.arrange(OR, lOR)
```

The asterisks denote significance (for `Broccoli` and `Age`). Notably, the 95% CI around the coefficient does not overlap the line of null effect (1 for odds ratios, 0 for log(odds)) for `Broccoli` and `Age`. Again, 95% CI must always be reported in

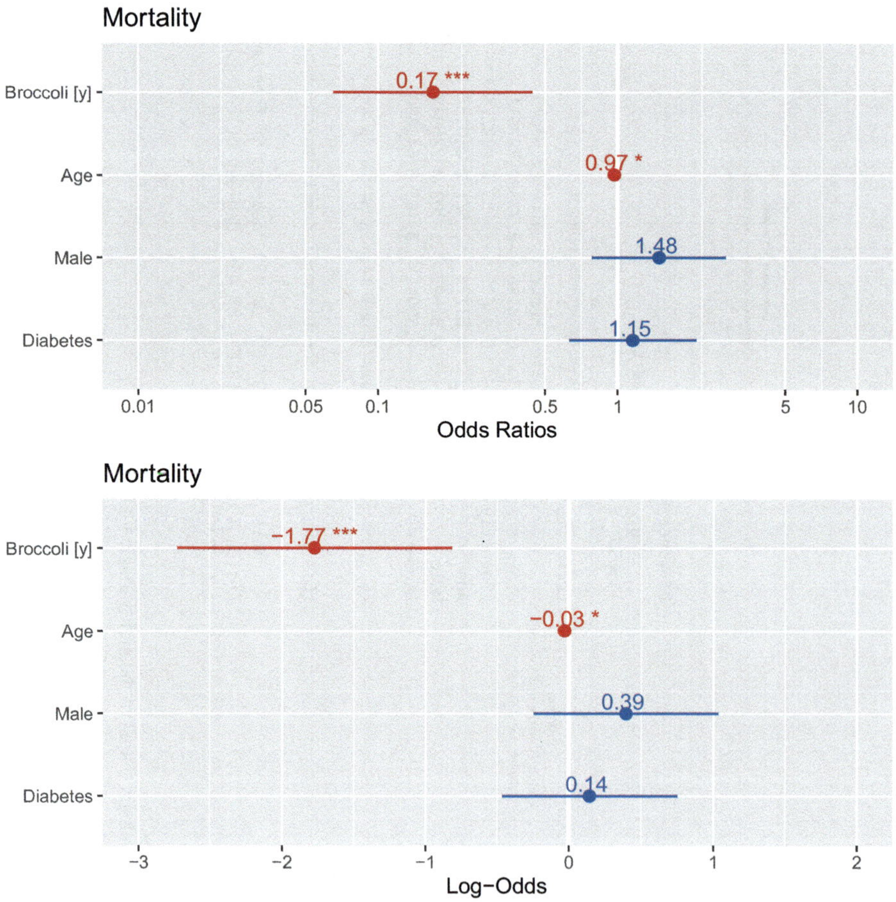

Fig. 10.13 Graphical depiction of odds ratio and log(odds) of the coefficients from multivariable logistic regression

	Mortality		
Predictors	*Odds Ratios*	*CI*	*p*
(Intercept)	0.76	0.17 – 3.16	0.708
Broccoli [y]	0.17	0.06 – 0.40	**<0.001**
Age	0.97	0.95 – 0.99	**0.010**
Male	1.48	0.78 – 2.83	0.227
Diabetes	1.15	0.60 – 2.04	0.642
Observations	500		

Fig. 10.14 Odds ratios with 95% confidence intervals

```
                OR  lower95ci upper95ci      Pr(>|Z|)
Broccoliy 0.1700215 0.06546537 0.4415663 0.0002740886
Age       0.9702628 0.94819091 0.9928484 0.0101322064
Male      1.4825965 0.78271190 2.8083031 0.2269443289
Diabetes  1.1547645 0.62968902 2.1176818 0.6418796751
```

Fig. 10.15 Odds ratios along with 95% confidence interval and p-values

a scientific paper. It can be obtained with many functions, one of them is `tab_model( )` (Fig. 10.14):

```
> tab_model(multimodel)
```

Similarly, we can use the `logistic.display( )` function as we did earlier in this chapter for simple logistic regression (Fig. 10.15).

```
> logistic.display(multimodel, alpha = 0.05, crude = FALSE,
crude.p.value = FALSE, decimal = 2, simplified = TRUE)
```

10.10 How Well the Regression Model Fits the Data?

It is mandatory to check the *performance* of the regression.

For logistic regression we should consider two approaches. The first is the *predictive power* of the model, and the second is the *goodness of fit* (GOF).

The predictive power of a model refers to how well the independent variables predict the dependent variable (also known as *explanatory power*). A prediction of *1* means that the explanatory variables predict the response variable completely. Vice versa, a prediction of *0* means no prediction at all. R-squared and the receiver operating characteristic (ROC) curve are a measure of prediction.

The GOF (model fit) is measured with the *Hosmer-Lemeshow statistic* and with *deviance*. Notably, those two approaches are unrelated. We can obtain a good model fit and yet very poor prediction from the same model.

10.11 R-Squared

R-squared is a value that spans from 0 to 1, where 0 is equal to the model explaining no variance/no predictive power, and 1 is equal to the model explaining all variance/strong predictive power.

We briefly looked at this test in Chap. 9 about linear regression.

In fact, for linear regression, because the outcome of interest is numeric, the R-squared calculation is specific, yet for logistic regression given the binary outcome we need a mathematical approximation. In logistic regression, R-squared is approximated by the McFadden (pseudo) R-squared test.

Let us calculate the McFadden (pseudo) R-squared test for the `multimodel` model. We use the `pscl` package and the `pR2` function (Fig. 10.16):

```
> pR2(multimodel)# the package pscl should be installed and loaded
```

Disappointingly, this value is very low. Careful interpretation is needed for R-squared and it also depends on the research field. While not necessarily low, R-squared undermines the model.

```
fitting null model for pseudo-r2
          llh       llhNull           G2     McFadden
-134.41129671 -148.94298418  29.06337493   0.09756544
         r2ML          r2CU
   0.05646965    0.12580597
```

Fig. 10.16 McFadden (pseudo) R-squared test

10.12 Area Under the ROC Curve (C-Statistic)

In statistics, *sensitivity* is "the probability that the model predicts a positive outcome for an observation when indeed the outcome is positive". This is also called the *true positive rate*.

In contrast, *specificity* is defined as "the probability that the model predicts a negative outcome for an observation when indeed the outcome is negative". This is also called the *true negative rate*.

One way to visualise these two metrics is by computing a ROC curve; ROC stands for *receiver operating characteristic*. The ROC curve (also known as c-statistic) is a plot that displays the sensitivity along the y-axis and (1- specificity) along the x-axis. In fact, ROC is a measure of *discrimination*, known as a "measure of how well the model can separate those who do and do not have the outcome of interest".

One way to quantify how well the logistic regression model does at classifying data is to calculate AUC, which is the *area under the curve*. The closer the AUC is to 1, the better the model. Let us go back to our multiple logistic regression `multimodel` model and compute the ROC curve along with the AUC. We will use the `ROCR` and `pROC` packages (Fig. 10.17).

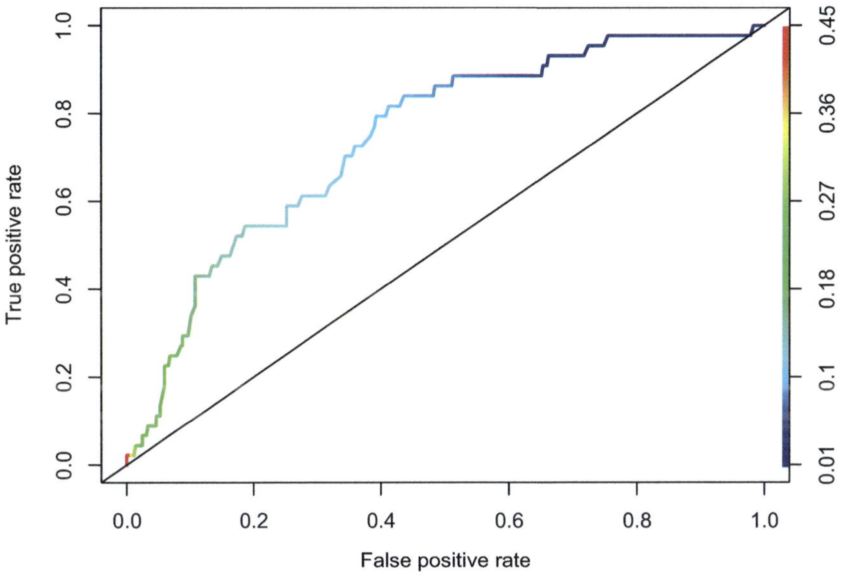

Fig. 10.17 ROC (c-statistic) for the multivariable multimodel model

```
> v<-c(predict(multimodel,type='response'))# creating the object
'v' with prediction values
> labels=MMstat$Mortality #Mortality is the dependent variable
> pred=prediction(v,labels)
> perf=performance(pred, 'tpr', 'fpr')# true positive rate, false
positive rate
> plot(perf, lwd=1, type='l', colorize=T)
> performance(pred, 'auc')
> abline(0, 1)
```

The AUC is calculated as below:

```
> predicted <- predict(multimodel, MMstat, type="response") #cal-
culate probability of default for each individual in test dataset
> auc(MMstat$Mortality, predicted) #calculate AUC
Area under the curve: 0.7437
```

with AUC of 0.74.

10.13 Deviance

This is a measure of GOF. Specifically, it is a measure of how the *prediction* differs from the *observed* outcome. Deviance ranges from 0 to infinity.

Again, in the context of linear regression, the deviance is easily calculated, since the outcome (dependent variable) can take any values, and we can measure how the predicted values differ from the observed outcome. In logistic regression this is not possible, since the observations in the outcome of interest can only be one of two levels (0 or 1), whereas the predicted values are computed with log(odds) and can be any value between 0 and 1. Some adjustments are required.

Let us calculate the *deviance*. This comes along with the `summary(multimodel)` function (Fig. 10.18):

"R" reports two types of deviance. The null deviance is the deviance of the model with intercept only. The residual deviance is obtained when we add our explanatory variables to the model (`Broccoli+Age+Male+Diabetes`), with an improvement (reduction) of deviance of 297.8 − 268.8 = 29. How can we interpret this reduction in deviance? What are the variables that effectively reduced the deviance in the model?

```
    Null deviance: 297.89  on 499  degrees of freedom
Residual deviance: 268.82  on 494  degrees of freedom
AIC: 280.82
```

Fig. 10.18 Deviance—the result is reported with the summary function

Again, the smaller the deviance the better. The `anova` function with `test = "Chisq"` tells what variables improved the model by reducing the deviance, starting from the null model (only intercept) to the proposed model, until the model saturates (Fig. 10.19):

```
> anova(multimodel, test = "Chisq")
```

The *p*-value in the last column on the right tells us that the deviance will only improve after adding `Broccoli` and `Age`, while adding `Male` and `Diabetes` will not improve the deviance.

Notably, the ANOVA function is also used as a way to compare a reduced nested model (simplified models with few variables) with the full model. This is also called *likelihood ratio test*. Let us consider a reduced model with only two variables and compare it to the full model as below (Fig. 10.20):

```
> reducedmodel<-glm(Mortality~Broccoli+Age,family='binomial'(link
=logit), data=MMstat)
> multimodel<-glm(Mortality~Broccoli+Age+Male+Diabetes,family='bi
nomial'(link=logit), data=MMstat)
> anova(reducedmodel, multimodel, test='Chisq')
```

In this case, there are no differences between the reduced model and the full model. Given that H0 holds that the reduced model is true, a p-value more than 0.05 for the overall model fit statistic would compel us to fail to reject the null

```
         Df Deviance Resid. Df Resid. Dev  Pr(>Chi)
NULL                       499     297.89
Broccoli  1  19.9805       498     277.90 7.823e-06 ***
Age       1   6.5185       497     271.39   0.01068 *
Male      1   1.4887       496     269.90   0.22242
Diabetes  2   1.0756       494     268.82   0.58402
---
```

Fig. 10.19 ANOVA function indicates which variable significantly reduces the deviance

```
Analysis of Deviance Table

Model 1: Mortality ~ Broccoli + Age
Model 2: Mortality ~ Broccoli + Age + Male + Diabetes
  Resid. Df Resid. Dev Df Deviance Pr(>Chi)
1       497     271.39
2       495     269.69  2   1.6976   0.4279
```

Fig. 10.20 Likelihood ratio test to compare nested model with full model

hypothesis. Hence, we should *prefer* the nested model that is a simplified version, since the full model does not add much to it.

10.14 AIC

This is short for *Akaike information criterion* (AIC) and measures the quality of a model in terms of the amount of information lost by that model. I also cover this topic in Chap. 9 on linear regression. The smaller the AIC the better. However, there is not an absolute value or a benchmark. AIC works as a way to compare models. As such a model with low AIC should be preferred. The AIC is returned within the `summary` function.

10.15 Hosmer-Lemeshow Statistic and Test

The Hosmer-Lemeshow test is computed on data after observations have been divided into certain groups (named as *g*) based on having *similar predicted probabilities*. It examines whether the observed proportions of events are similar to the predicted probabilities of occurrence in subgroups of the dataset, using Pearson's chi-squared test.

There is little guidance as to how to choose the number of groups within *g*. Hosmer and Lemeshow's conclusions from simulations were based on using $g > p+1$, suggesting that if we have 10 covariates in the model, we should choose $g > 11$. We must load the `ResourceSelection` library (Fig. 10.21).

```
> hl <- hoslem.test(multimodel$y, fitted(multimodel), g=5) #Hosmer-
Lemeshow test, library(ResourceSelection), we choose g =5 since we
have 4 covariates in the model
> hl
```

The null hypothesis holds that the model fits the data (high values are best). In our case the p-value associated with our model is 0.75.

```
        Hosmer and Lemeshow goodness of fit (GOF) test

data:  multimodel$y, fitted(multimodel)
X-squared = 1.2069, df = 3, p-value = 0.7513
```

Fig. 10.21 Hosmer and Lemeshow's goodness of fit test

10.16 Overfitting

Overfitting is a statistical hazard that can potentially affect every regression model. There is a *theoretical limited space* in every model; in fact only a limited number of explanatory variables can be accommodated.

Categorical variables with many levels are very cumbersome and occupy a large space in the model. Linear variables or categorical variables with only two levels are less heavy. When the model is forced with too many variables, it becomes overinflated and unstable.

The capacity of the model to accommodate the explanatory variables depends on its sample size.

"R" tells us when there is overfitting. It returns the warning of *no convergence*, indicating that the software did not find the algorithm to literally juggle all the explanatory variables.

Nevertheless, even if the algorithm converged, there could still be overfitting. It is pivotal to double check the size of the ORs and their standard error. Vast and spread numbers with large confidence intervals are signs of overfitting. Standard error above 1 may already indicate overfitting.

Overfitting is most common for logistic regression rather than linear regression. It may also happen when covariates are highly correlated.

Ultimately the aim is to build and achieve a model that is *robust* and can be exported to other datasets leading to the same results.

10.17 Variance Inflation Factor

As we did for linear regression in Chap. 9, we can use the variance inflation factor (VIF) as a diagnostic tool for multicollinearity. It is named variance inflation factor since it estimates how much the variance of a coefficient is *inflated*.

VIF has a lower bound of 1 with no upper limit. A VIF of 1.6 means that the variance of that particular coefficient is 60% larger than it would be if that predictor was completely non-correlated to the others. To check for collinearity we use the `rms` package. As before, we use the `vif` function (Fig. 10.22).

Let us consider this model:

```
> library(rms)#we need this library
> vif(multimodel)
      Age       bmi        CC       CPB  Bleeding      LVEF
 1.113564  1.022261  2.072381  4.663676  4.023381  1.036920
Broccoliy   Aspirin      Male  Diabetes
 1.050020  1.177030  1.016406  1.026894
> plot_model(multimodel, type='diag')
```

Generally, VIF lower than 5 does not affect the beta regression coefficient. In our model composed of three explanatory variables, no significant VIF was detected.

```
> library(rms)#we need this library
> vif(multimodel)
      Age       bmi        CC       CPB  Bleeding      LVEF
 1.113564  1.022261  2.072381  4.663676  4.023381  1.036920
Broccoliy   Aspirin      Male  Diabetes
 1.050020  1.177030  1.016406  1.026894
> plot_model(multimodel, type='diag')
```

Fig. 10.22 Variance inflation factors

10.18 Conclusions

Models do not reproduce or exactly imitate *life*; rather they *approximate* life. This is the aim of regression (both linear and logistic), and once again all models are wrong but some of them are useful. When the outcome of interest is binary, we use logistic regression. Notably, logistic regression is also part of the machine learning techniques, since it is a classification method. Rather than measuring directly the value of the dependent variable, we use logistic regression, because we are interested in the probability of the event occurring given certain explanatory variables. To perform logistic regression, we need to transform the y-value that is confined to 0 or 1, to log(odds). The latter can take any number, from negative infinite to positive infinite. By exponentiating the log(odds) we obtain the odds ratios. As per linear regression, a model with only one explanatory variable is a simple model, while a model with many explanatory variables is a multiple model (multiple logistic regression). Logistic regression can handle both numeric and non-numeric explanatory variables, as shown in examples throughout this chapter. Some assumptions must hold, such as linearity between the continuous explanatory variable and the log(odds) of the dependent variables.

The model built from our `MMstat` dataset is undermined by the scarcity of `Mortality` events; hence, only a few explanatory variables were considered in the final model.

Finally, I explained how to check prediction power and goodness of fit of the model.

Further Readings

Bruce P, Bruce A. Practical statistics for data scientists. Sebastopol, CA: O'Reilly Media; 2017.
Hosmer D, Lemeshow S. Applied logistic regression. 2nd ed. New York: Wiley; 2000.
James G, Witten D, Hastie T, Tibshirani R. An introduction to statistical learning: with applications in R. New York: Springer Publishing Company; 2014.

Long JS, Freese J. Regression models for categorical dependent variables using Stata. 2nd ed. College Station, TX: Stata Press; 2006.

Mittlböck M, Schemper M. Explained variation for logistic regression. Stat Med. 1996;15(19):1987–97.

Chapter 11
Time-to-Event Analysis

Time-to-Event Analysis

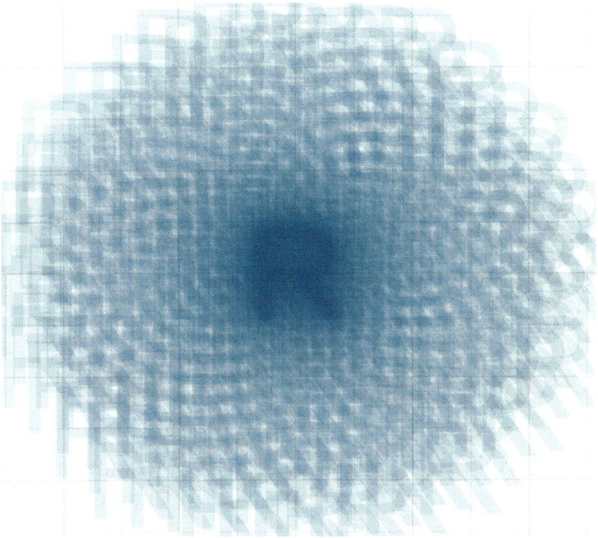

This chapter reviews and teaches the basics of survival analysis using "R". It does this by analysing our example dataset, to understand whether there are differences in survival between the two groups of patients, those who included `Broccoli` before cardiac surgery and those who did not. It also shows you how to apply Cox regression to explore independent predictors for a specific outcome at follow-up.

M. Moscarelli, *Biostatistics With 'R': A Guide for Medical Doctors*,
https://doi.org/10.1007/978-3-031-33073-5_11

11.1 Software and R-Packages Required for This Chapter

If you haven't already, you need to download and install base-R and R-studio as set out in Chap. 2 under the heading "Downloading "R" and R-studio".

The relevant R-packages needed for this chapter are:

- Survival—it can be downloaded at:
- https://github.com/therneau/survival
- Survminer—it can be downloaded at:
- http://www.sthda.com/english/rpkgs/survminer

11.2 Where to Download the Example Dataset and Script for This Chapter

If you haven't already downloaded the supplementary dataset named `MMstat.csv` created as a practical example for use throughout this book, you will find it at the link that follows. The script for this chapter named `Chapter 11.Time to event.R` can also be found and downloaded at the following link:

https://github.com/mmlondon77/Biobook.git.

11.3 Time-to-Event Analysis

How long before a certain event of interest occurs? For example, how long before a cancer relapse or re-hospitalisation occurs? These examples can be handled with *time-to-event* analysis.

There are countless types of events or outcomes. When the event of interest is *death*, the time-to-event analysis is named *survival analysis*. Ultimately, time-to-event analysis and survival analysis indicate the same statistical technique; it is just the nature of the event that is different.

Let us return to our `MMstat` dataset. As part of the research question, we may want to investigate if the group of patients who included `Broccoli` before surgery survived longer than those who did not. Perhaps there was no difference. Perhaps the `noBroccoli` group in fact lived longer than the `Broccoli` group. Perhaps we have just one group, and we are simply interested in survival after a certain exposure to treatment.

In our specific time-to-event analysis, the event of interest (defined as a binary event) is *death*. As I said, every event of a binary nature can be analysed by the aims of time-to-event analysis. This is similar to logistic regression, where the outcome of interest is also binary. However, the statistical technique here is different, since in time-to-event analysis we have also a continuous variable to handle, being *time* (the time until the event occurs). In logistic regression we are in fact interested in whether or not the outcome or event happened, rather than *when*. On the contrary, in time-to-event analysis we are interested in *how long it takes for the event or outcome to occur*.

You may have noticed that we are using interchangeable outcomes or events.

Our event of interest should be *unambiguous*, *clinically relevant*, *well defined* and *easily observable*. While *death* may seem unambiguous, misclassification is possible when a specific cause of death is the outcome of interest. In fact, in medicine we are quite often interested in cardiovascular or cancer mortality. We must be very explicit in terms of mortality adjudication (i.e. how did the patient die? Was it cancer, cardiovascular causes, a car accident, etc.).

With regard to cancer, we should also specify the time of diagnosis, rather than the time of occurrence, since they do not occur instantaneously. In this context, we would better refer to *time-to-diagnosis*. Survival analysis in cancer screening studies can be misleading since it depends on when the disease was diagnosed. Observed prolonged survival time could be related only due to the disease being diagnosed at an early stage and may not necessarily reflect absolute survival time.

There are some key aspects that constitute survival/time-to-event analysis. They are:

- Censoring
- Survival function, Kaplan-Meier and log-rank test
- Hazard function
- Cox regression
- Analysis of the residuals to check the proportional hazard function assumptions

11.4 Censoring

Time-to-event analysis focuses on the expected duration of time until a certain binary event occurs (i.e. death, cancer relapse, etc.). However, for whatever reason, such an event may not be observed during the period of time of analysis. An example of this could be an individual does not experience the event of interest, then perhaps is lost at follow-up. Those individuals are considered *censored*.

Right censoring is the most common type of censoring. To explain what right censoring is, I refer back to our research question. We are interested in the survival rates of patients who undergo surgery and who are also split into two groups, one group including a broccoli dietary regime before surgery vs another group who ate a liberal diet prior to surgery. Importantly, we know exactly the dates (day, month, year) of their operations. Thereby, we track the patients from the known day of their operations (*time origin*) to the moment of our last follow-up (*end of study*).

Let us consider Fig. 11.1, with ten patients (called *at risk*) enrolled in a study and all of them at a certain point in the future, during the period of observation, experience the event of interest (death):

In this example, with a follow-up of 10 months, we have no censoring, because the event occurred in all patients before the end of the study. Every month, one participant experiences an event. After every month, the survival probability drops by 10% *of the remaining curve*. That's because we need to divide the number of events by the patients at risk, which in this case is (1/10 = 0.1 = 10%). For example, at time equals 2 months, we have another event, and the curve drops by 10% of the remaining curve (overall 20%). Eventually the curve reaches the zero value with 10 events. I will talk about survival probability soon. But what happens if a patient does not experience the event until the study has ended? In other words, what if we have censored patients?

Censored patients are normally indicated with the + symbol. They are most often coded as `0` opposed to `1`, whereby `0` indicates that the event occurs.

Censored individuals are not counted as the event having occurred even if we lose contact with them (i.e. lost at follow-up); hence, they are considered as non-informative (censoring is never caused by the *event* that defines the endpoint of the study). However, they are removed from the overall count of patients at risk. Let us consider Fig. 11.2:

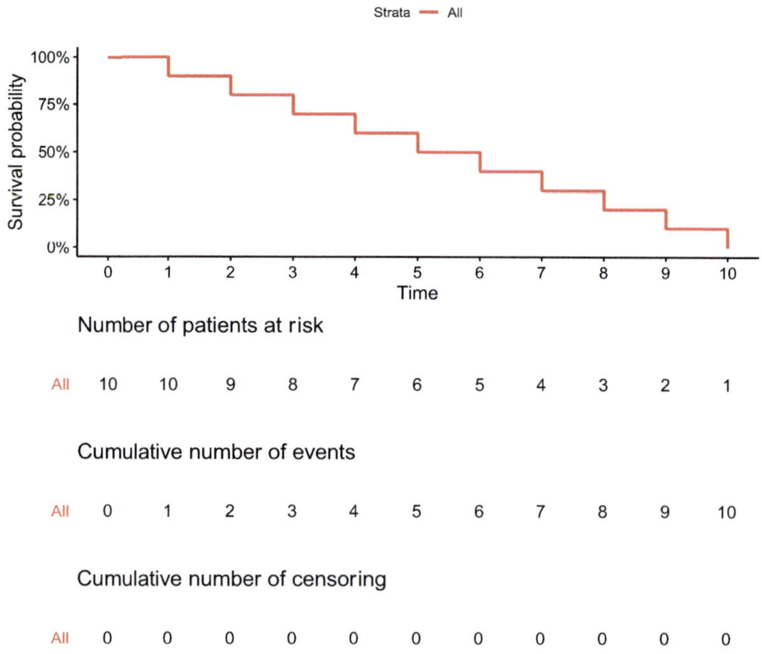

Fig. 11.1 Time-to-event analysis

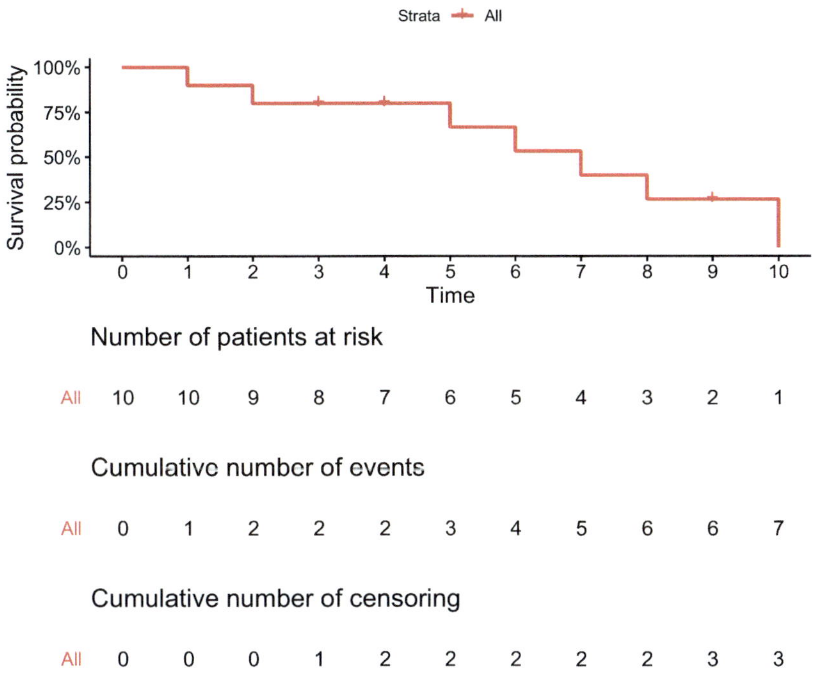

Fig. 11.2 Survival analysis plotted with Kaplan-Meier

With regard to the first 2 months, this plot looks similar to the previous one with no censoring, with a drop of 10% for the step. Yet after the second month (3rd and 4th months) we have two censored patients, and at 5 months we have an event. Now the denominator of the patients at risk changes; we have two events and two censored patients, and the drop of the curve (the step) is not anymore 1 out of 10 (10%) but instead 1 out of 6 (16% of the remaining height, hence a bigger step than before). I will demonstrate how to calculate *survival tables* with both censored and no censored patients in the next paragraphs.

In my opinion, it is important to plot the curve (as I did in Figs. 11.1 and 11.2) along with three factors:

1. Number of patients at risk
2. Number of events
3. Number of censored (no events or lost at follow-up)

These practical examples are based only on ten patients. The curves are also presented with 95% confidence intervals. It goes without saying that a small study has a large 95% confidence interval. The more we move to the right side of the curve, the more uncertainty we have, since fewer patients survived.

11.5 Other Types of Censoring

Right censoring technique is the most common type of censoring and widely used in medicine. There are other types of censoring, such as left censoring and interval censoring. Those however will not be covered in this chapter, since they are rarely used in medicine.

Briefly, *left censoring* occurs when we know that the individual experienced the event before the start of the observation, but the exact time of the event is unknown (i.e. unknown time of origin). *Interval censoring* is similar to left censoring; however, it is known that the event occurred between two specific time points, yet again the exact time of origin is unknown.

11.6 Survival Function, Kaplan-Meier and Log-Rank Test

The survival function is merely the probability that an individual survives up to and including the time *t*, or in the context of a time-to-event analysis, the probability that the event of interest (i.e. cancer relapse) does not occur up to and including the time *t*:

$$S(t) = \Pr(T > t)$$

whereby T is the time of death (or of the event of interest) and $\Pr(T > t)$ is the probability that the time of the event is greater than time t. S is a probability:

$$0 \leq S(t) \leq 1$$

And survival times are always positive:

$$T \geq 0$$

Notably, survival analysis deals with *time*, hence with positive values more often right skewed. For example, linear models assume normal distribution, not appropriate for positive outcomes. This is another reason why linear models do not handle time-to-event analysis.

Kaplan-Meier (KM) is a non-parametric method that *illustrates* survival function (i.e. KM plots survival function!). Again, no assumption is made about the underlying distribution (e.g. normality). However, there are some other general assumptions that need to be in place.

Firstly, at any time, patients who are censored have the same survival prospects as those who continue to be followed.

Secondly, survival probabilities are the same for subjects recruited in the early and the late period of the study.

Lastly, the events of interest happen precisely at the time specified.

In the previous figures we have seen that Kaplan-Meier is a *step* function which illustrates cumulative survival over time.

The survival probability at any specific time point is calculated by the formula below:

$$\text{St} = \frac{\text{Overall number of subjetcs at risk} - \text{Number of subject with the events}}{\text{Overall number of subjetcs at risk}}$$

This fares well in the hypothetical and unrealistic scenario of no *censored patients*, when all the patients experienced the event/outcome of interest before the end of the study. The scenario set out in Fig. 11.1 is a good example of this, whereby for 10 patients followed up for 10 months, the event occurs at a certain point for all of them (1 event each month), and the survival probability, let's say at 5 months, is 10-5/10 = 50%:

$$\text{St} = \frac{10-5}{10}$$

However, when we have censored patients, both numerator and denominator change and the probability of surviving past day t is simply the probability of surviving past day $t - 1$ multiplied by the proportion of patients that survive on day t. To better explain, let us analyse the second scenario, which includes censored patients (Table 11.1).

We have censored patients at time=3 and time=4 (indicated with the symbol +). This now means the count of patients at risk is n=10 *minus* the cumulative number of events (2) and *minus* the number of censored patients (2). Hence, when we calculate the proportion of patients surviving past time=5, we should take into account a survival basket of patients at risk, being $n = 6$ (no longer $n = 10$). The survival probability past time t=5 is then calculated multiplying the probability of $t - 1 * t$ (0.80*0.83=0.66%).

Table 11.1

Time (t) days	Number of patients alive at time t	Number of patients who died at time t	Proportion of patients surviving past time t	Survival probability past time t
1	10	1	(10 – 1)/10 = 0.9	0.90 (90%)
2 ++	9	1	(9 – 1)/9 = 0.88	0.90*0.88 = 0.80
5	6	1	(6 – 1)/6 = 0.83	0.80*0.83 = 0.66
6	5	1	(5 – 1)/5 = 0.8	0.66*0.80 = 0.53
7	4	1	(4 – 1)/4 = 0.75	0.52*0.75 = 0.40
8+	3	1	(3 – 1)/3 = 0.66	0.40*0.66 = 0.26
10	1	1	0	0

11.7 Log-Rank Test

Let us compare two survival curves with Kaplan-Meier below. From the curves we can compare, at certain given time points, the survival probability between group 1 and group 2, but we cannot tell if there is a difference at all (Fig. 11.3).

Log-rank takes the entire follow-up period into account.

The log-rank test is used to test the null hypothesis, being that there is no difference in the probability of an event (i.e. death) between the two populations of interest (i.e. broccoli vs no-broccoli, or group 1 and group 2) at any time point within the study period.

It is a non-parametric test, with no assumption of the underlying distribution. It shares the same assumptions as the Kaplan-Meier survival curves.

Importantly, while log-rank tells us if there are significant differences, it does not say anything about the magnitude of the difference. We should also note that the log-rank test is most likely to detect differences between groups, when the risk of an event is consistently greater for one group than the other. Nevertheless, it is the most used test in survival analysis for comparing two groups.

One particular case scenario is when the two curves cross, as a result of the survival times having greater variance in one treatment group than the other. Therefore, log-rank should not be used. We will in fact see that the hazard proportion (the risk) between the two groups should be constant at any point, with no interaction with time. We explore this situation further when we examine residuals later in this chapter.

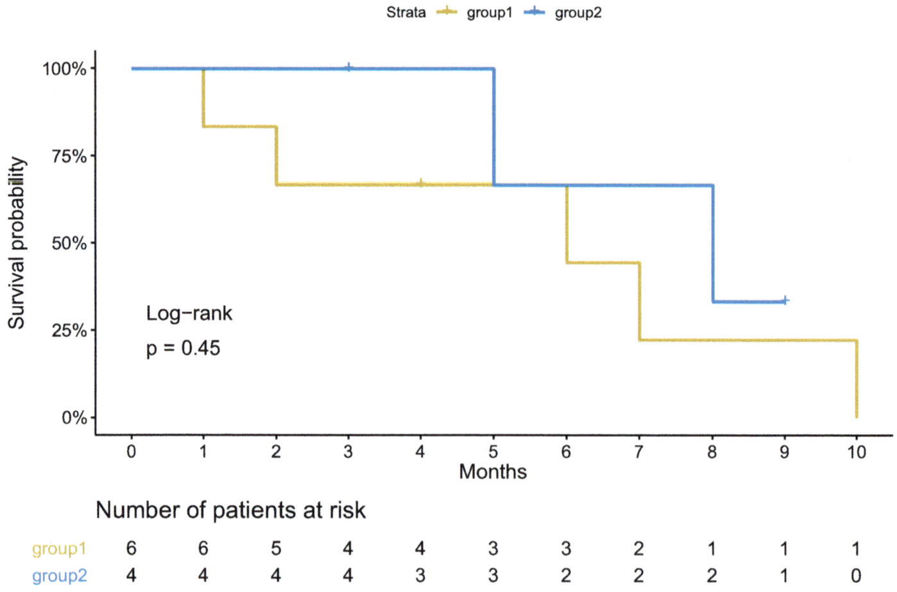

Fig. 11.3 Survival analysis with two groups and log-rank test

11.8 Hazard Function

Sometimes in medicine, survival data is presented by the aim of *hazard function* rather than survival function.

Hazard function, denoted as $h(t)$, can be interpreted as the reverse of the survival function and is an expression of risk in a certain period. It is the probability that a certain individual who is under observation at a given time t experiences the event at that time.

It is very easy in "R" to plot survival as hazard function. I provide the code soon in this chapter. For the moment, I provide an example of how hazard function looks (Fig. 11.4):

As already stated, it is pivotal to understand that survival analysis does not assume that hazard is constant. For example, the hazard straight after surgery is higher, and it can also increase with age. However, it does assume that the ratio of hazards between groups is constant over time.

As a reminder:

- Hazard ratio (HR) = 1: no effect
- Hazard ratio (HR) > 1: increase in hazard
- Hazard ratio (HR) < 1: decrease in hazard

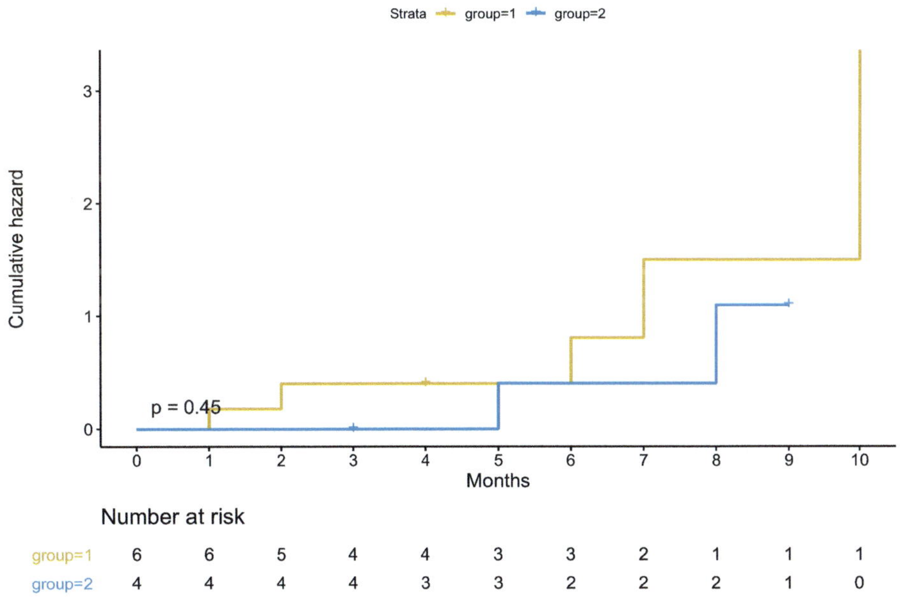

Fig. 11.4 Hazard function

11.9 Survival Probability in Our Dataset

Before moving to Cox regression to explore which covariates are independently associated to our outcome of interest at follow-up, we can draw survival curves using our `MMstat` dataset, taking into account two groups: `Broccoli=y` and `Broccoli=n`.

We may want to exclude early post-operative mortality and only include the patients who survived after 30 days. We normally apply logistic regression to understand which covariates would influence the post-operative mortality (i.e. 30-day mortality).

```
mmstat<-MMstat[MMstat$Mortality=='0',]#selecting the patients who
survived the operation
View(mmstat)
```

To plot the survival probability with Kaplan-Meier I use the `survival` package and the `survfit( )` function:

```
> library(survival)
> myfit <- survfit(Surv(FUtime, FUmortality) ~ 1, type='kaplan-
meier', data = mmstat)#null model, creating the object 'myfit',
specifying the time of death at follow up ('FUtime') and when the
patient died ('FUmortality'),in our case in months. Lastly, I need
to specify that I am interested in whether the patients died or not
(0/1), given by the symbol '~ 1'
```

Note that with the code above I plot the overall group. Before analysing the life table (survival probability at given time points), let us plot the results (*graphics bring data to life!*). For this we use the `survminer` package and the `ggsurvplot( )` function (Fig. 11.5):

```
> ggsurvplot(myfit, linetype=1, conf.int = TRUE, xlim=c(0,25),
ylim=c(0.9,1),risk.table = TRUE,tables.theme=theme_
cleantable(),risk.table.title='Number of patients at risk',
tables.height=0.18, surv.scale='percent', xlab='Months')
```

The survival probability is now plotted as a step function with Kaplan-Meier. Note that to amplify the curve, I rescaled the y-axis, to *zoom in*. It now goes from 90 to 100%.

The associated life table can be obtained with (Fig. 11.6):

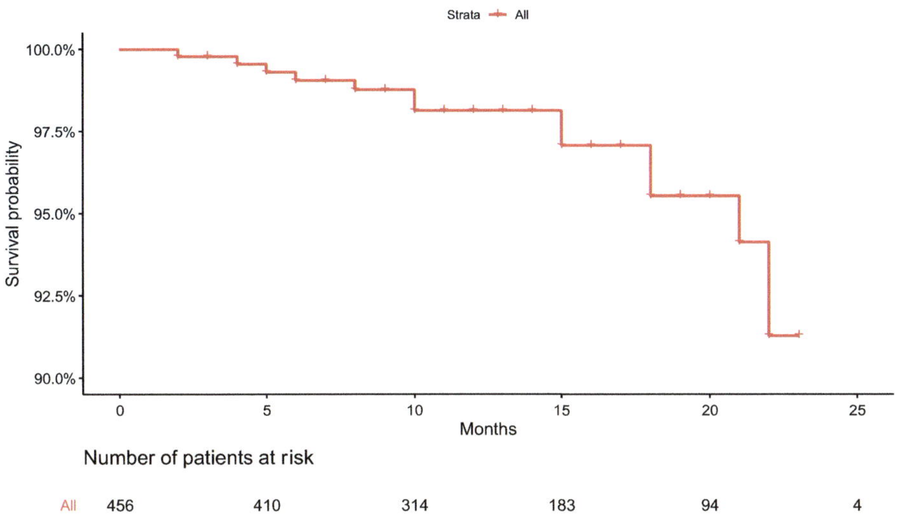

Fig. 11.5 Survival probability, overall cohort

```
Call: survfit(formula = Surv(FUtime, FUmortality) ~ 1, data = mmstat,
    type = "kaplan-meier")

 time n.risk n.event survival std.err lower 95% CI upper 95% CI
    5    410       3    0.993 0.00399        0.985        1.000
   10    314       4    0.981 0.00702        0.968        0.995
   15    183       2    0.971 0.01025        0.951        0.991
   20     94       2    0.955 0.01472        0.927        0.985
```

Fig. 11.6 Survival probability at different time

```
> summary(myfit, time=c(5,10,15,20))#life table
```

As can be seen from Fig. 11.6, in the overall cohort, survival at 15 months is 97%, with a 95% confidence interval of 95% to 99%.

Before adding the categorical `Broccoli` variable, I think it is important to discuss *median survival time*, very often found in survival analysis. First, I should say that survival times are not normally distributed, so mean is not an appropriate summary, and hence the median is computed. The median survival is the time corresponding to a survival probability of 0.5 (50%). Interestingly, according to our sample size, we cannot compute the median since the cohort *has not yet dropped to 50% survival* at the end of the available data. Therefore, there would be NA values for median survival.

Let us verify with the following function (Fig. 11.7):

```
Call: survfit(formula = Surv(FUtime, FUmortality) ~ 1, data = mmstat,
    type = "kaplan-meier")

      n  events  median 0.95LCL 0.95UCL
    456      14      NA      NA      NA
```

Fig. 11.7 Evaluating the median follow-up

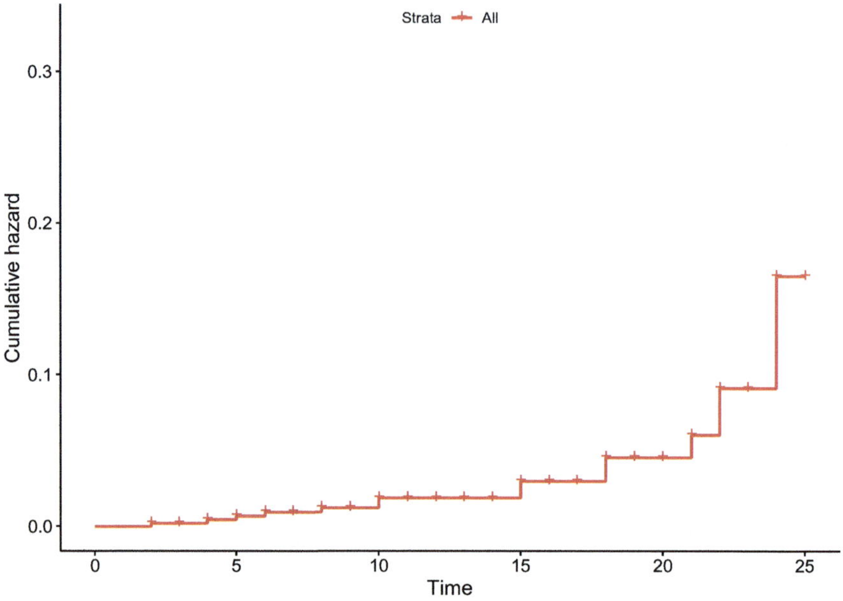

Fig. 11.8 Cumulative hazard function

```
> print(myfit)
```

As you can see in Fig. 11.7, "R" is in fact returning `NA` values, because it is not possible to calculate the median survival.

Importantly, to obtain the hazard function we should specify the `fun='cumhaz'` function (Fig. 11.8):

```
> ggsurvplot(myfit, fun='cumhaz')
```

11.10 Adding Categorical *Broccoli* Variable

Say at this point, we would like to plot the survival probability of the two groups, `Broccoli=='y'` and `Broccoli=='n'`:

```
> Bfit <- survfit(Surv(FUtime, FUmortality) ~ Broccoli, data = mmstat)
> ggsurvplot(Bfit, linetype=1,  pval = TRUE, pval.method=TRUE,
conf.int = TRUE, surv.median.line='hv',xlim=c(0,25),risk.table
=TRUE, tables.theme=theme_cleantable(), risk.table.title='Number
of patients at risk',tables.height=0.18, surv.scale='percent',
legend.labs = c("noBroccoli","Broccoli"), xlab='Months', palette
= c("#E7B800", "#2E9FDF"))
```

From Fig. 11.9 we can see that both survival curves look similar. The log-rank is obtained by specifying `pval = TRUE`. Note that the median survival is not returned even after I specified to plot it using `surv.median.line='hv'`; again this is because the 50% survival mark was not reached.

Finally, let's produce a life table:

```
> summary(Bfit, time=c(5,10,15,20))#life table
```

From Fig. 11.10, we can now tell that at 15 months the survival probability was 96% (95% CI = 94%, 99%) vs 97% (95% CI = 94%, 100%), for `Broccoli=='N'` and `Broccoli=='Y'`, respectively. The log-rank p-value test is 0.74; we can't reject the null (there is no difference between the two groups). We can conclude that survival probability does not differ in the two groups.

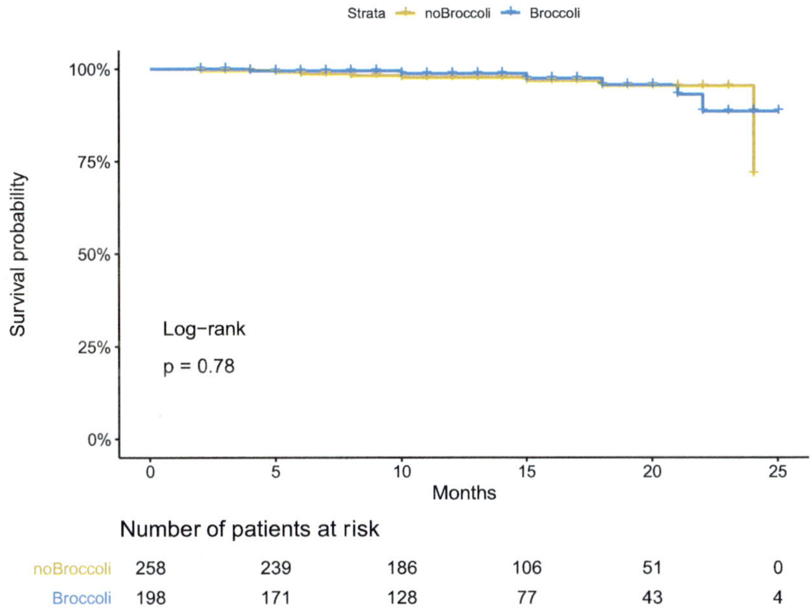

Fig. 11.9 Kaplan-Meier plotting survival analysis for two groups and log-rank test

```
Call: survfit(formula = Surv(FUtime, FUmortality) ~ Broccoli, data = mmstat)

                Broccoli=n
 time n.risk n.event survival std.err lower 95% CI upper 95% CI
    5    239       2    0.992 0.00567        0.981        1.000
   10    186       3    0.978 0.00993        0.958        0.997
   15    106       1    0.968 0.01345        0.942        0.995
   20     51       1    0.955 0.01909        0.918        0.993

                Broccoli=y
 time n.risk n.event survival std.err lower 95% CI upper 95% CI
    5    171       1    0.995 0.00545        0.984            1
   10    128       1    0.987 0.00944        0.968            1
   15     77       1    0.974 0.01578        0.944            1
   20     43       1    0.957 0.02296        0.913            1
```

Fig. 11.10 Life table

11.11 Cox Proportional Hazard (PH) Model (Cox Regression)

Cox regression is named after the British statistician David Cox and is the basis of survival analysis. What is the difference between log-rank, Kaplan-Meier and Cox regression? While log-rank can handle just one predictor, Cox regression (also better known as *Cox proportional hazard model*) can handle one predictor or *many* predictors. It is in fact conceptually similar to regression.

Also, log-rank does not provide the magnitude of the effect, it provides only a p-value.

Differently from Kaplan-Meier, Cox regression is a semi-parametric model.

In statistics, *hazard* is a risk of death (or the risk of the outcome of interest occurring) at a given moment in time. *Hazard ratio* is the ratio between two *hazard rates*. It is similar to odds ratio for logistic regression (except the underlying math is different).

Cox proportional hazard model has some specifications. By definition, the hazards assumed by the model must be *proportional*; they don't change with time.

Here is the algebraic formula for Cox regression:

$$h(t|X_i) = h_0(t)\exp\left(\beta_1 X_{i1} + \ldots \beta_{1p} X_{ip}\right)$$

Let's produce a simple Cox regression model with one predictor (the `Broccoli` variable), using the `coxph( )` function:

```
> coxfit<-coxph(Surv(FUtime, FUmortality) ~ Broccoli, data=mmstat)
> summary(coxfit)
```

The summary in Fig. 11.11 returns many interesting numbers, such as the HR with the standard error (se), 95% confidence interval, the associated p-value and also other indicators of model performance such as concordance, likelihood ratio test, Wald test and score log-rank.

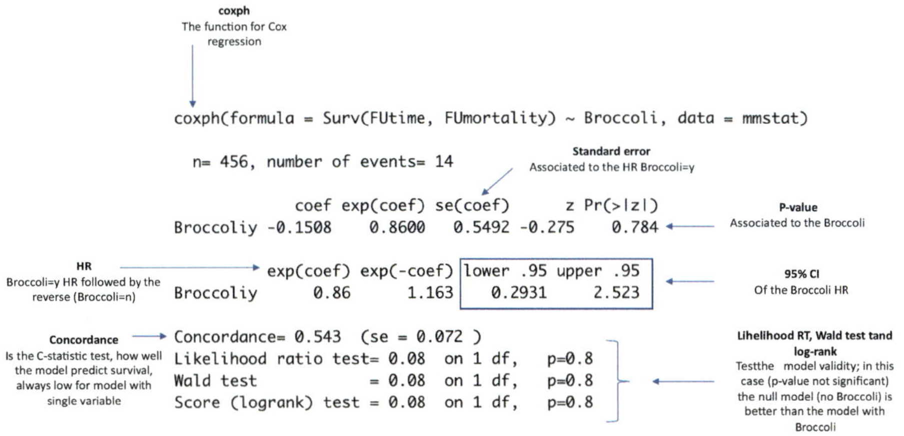

Fig. 11.11 Cox regression interpretation

Concordance tells how well the model predicts survival. It is similar to discrimination of C statistic. With just one covariate (`Broccoli`) concordance may be low (i.e. 0.5 equals to 50/50, hence low prediction).

Likelihood ratio, Wald and score log-rank all test whether to accept or reject the null hypothesis, which is *the model with* `Broccoli` *is not better than without* `Broccoli`. In this case we cannot reject the null (statistically the model with `Broccoli` is not better than the model without `Broccoli`).

These three tests will tend to be asymptotically similar with large sample size. With relatively low samples, score log-rank performs best.

The output returns coefficients with no intercepts because it is a semi-parametric model. From this simple Cox regression analysis, we can conclude that `Broccoli` does not affect mortality ($p = 0.78$). We knew that from the log-rank statistic, but now we also have an HR (expression of magnitude) of 0.86 with 95% CI: 0.29, 2.5.

A multiple Cox regression model is just an extension of a simple regression model to incorporate multiple predictors.

11.12 Analysis of the Residuals

How do I know if my model of Cox regression has a good performance? The lesson from linear regression tells us that we need to check the residuals. There are three types of residuals that we need to check in Cox regression, and those are:

1. *Schoenfeld residuals*: test whether two hazard functions are parallel or proportional. For example, when we plot the hazard for the broccoli group (a given predictor), it should be more or less parallel to the no-broccoli group (hazard should be proportional for a given predictor). We can then multiply the

hazard for the broccoli group and obtain the hazard for the no-broccoli group at any point in time.

If they do not correlate with time and are therefore *independent of time* with random pattern, then the assumption is valid. A residual test is good with a high *p*-value (testing for non-zero slope).

2. *Martingale residuals*: test whether a continuous predictor (e.g. CPB from the `MMstat` dataset) has a linear relationship with the outcome, or whether we need to add more terms to the model (e.g. CPB squared). Martingale residuals have a mean of zero, so values near 1 represent patients who died earlier than predicted, whereas large negative values represent patients who died later than predicted. The resulting plot should give you a nice straight line if the assumption is valid.
3. *Deviance residuals*: are used to spot influential points. These are data points that are unusual enough to have a big influence on the coefficients.

11.13 How to Calculate Schoenfeld Residuals

This is the most common test for testing proportionality assumptions. We can test it graphically and numerically (*p*-value). If the value is above 0.05, there is no strong evidence against a hazard proportionality assumption (i.e. there is no interaction between covariates of interest and time). Let's consider a multiple Cox model with four (`Broccoli+Male+Age+Bleeding`) covariates. To do so, we use the `cox.zph( )` function:

```
> multifit <- coxph(Surv(FUtime, FUmortality) ~
Broccoli+Male+Age+Bleeding, data=mmstat)
> temp <- cox.zph(multifit)
> print(temp)
```

As we see in Fig. 11.12, since all the p-values are above the significant level, there is no significant evidence against proportionality violation. Let's plot it with the `ggcoxzph( )` function (Fig. 11.13):

Fig. 11.12 Calculating the Schoenfeld residuals

```
         chisq df    p
Broccoli 0.163  1 0.69
Male     0.125  1 0.72
Age      1.024  1 0.31
Bleeding 1.385  1 0.24
GLOBAL   2.245  4 0.69
```

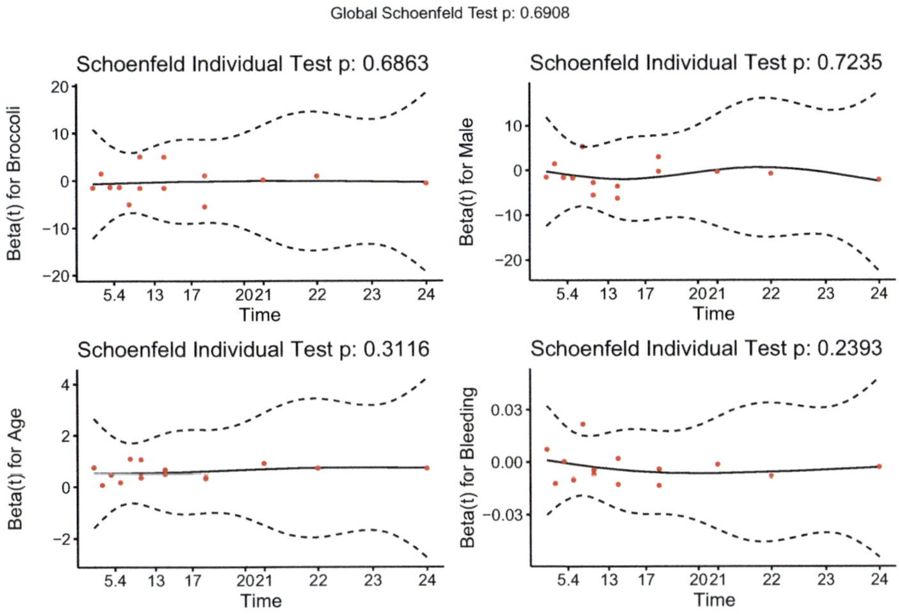

Fig. 11.13 Schoenfeld global and individual test

```
> ggcoxzph(temp)
```

From Fig. 11.13, the solid lines are the smoothing spline fit for each plot, with the dashed lines representing a ±2 standard error band around the fit. The null hypothesis is that the slope is equal to 0. We can observe a straight solid line which may suggest that the proportional assumption is met.

11.14 How to Calculate Martingale Residuals

We can visualise the Martingale residual with the `ggcoxdiagnostics( )` function specifying `type = "dfbeta"` (Fig. 11.14):

```
> ggcoxdiagnostics(multifit, type = "dfbeta", linear.predictions =
FALSE, ggtheme = theme_bw())
```

Again, values near 1 represent patients who died earlier than predicted; on the contrary negative values represent patients who died later than predicted. The resulting plot should return a straight line if the assumption is valid.

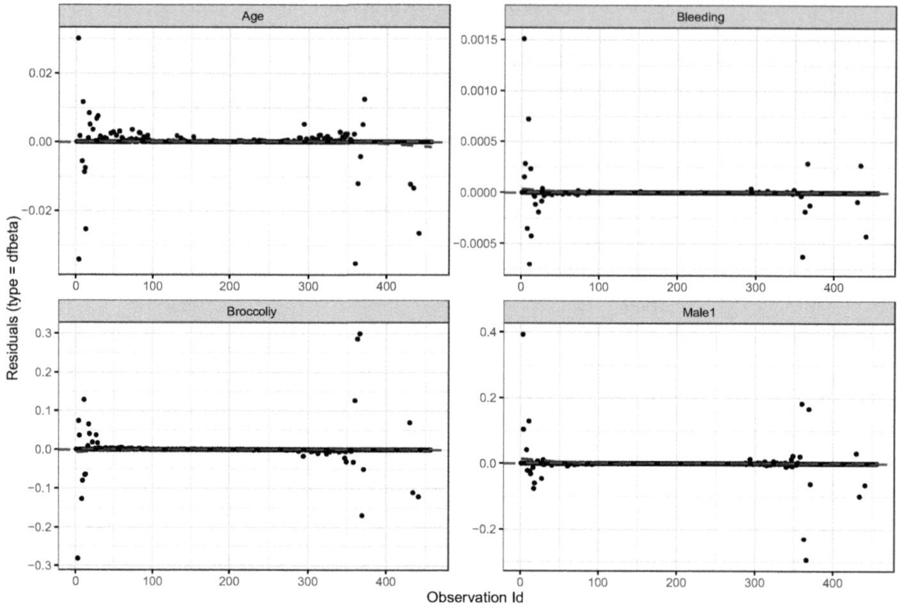

Fig. 11.14 Martingale residuals

11.15 Deviance Residuals

It is also possible to check outliers by visualising the deviance residuals, which are normalised transformations of the Martingale residuals and should be roughly symmetrically distributed about zero with a standard deviation of 1 (Fig. 11.15):

```
> ggcoxdiagnostics(multifit, type = "deviance", linear.predictions
= FALSE, ggtheme = theme_bw())
```

Another issue is whether any continuous variables that are assumed to have a linear relationship with the outcome actually do have a linear relationship. If you fit `CPB` as a single term in the model, then that's what you're assuming. The Martingale residual is used to test this assumption:

```
> ggcoxfunctional(Surv(FUtime, FUmortality) ~ CPB + log(CPB) +
sqrt(CPB), data=mmstat)
```

If the assumption is valid the plots should give you nice straight lines. However, looking at Fig. 11.16, there are problems with linearity.

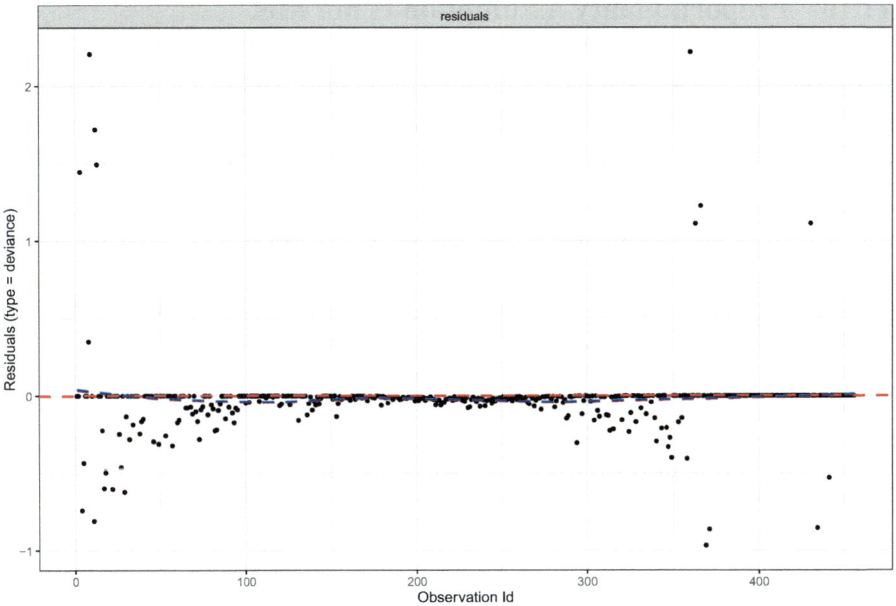

Fig. 11.15 Deviance residuals

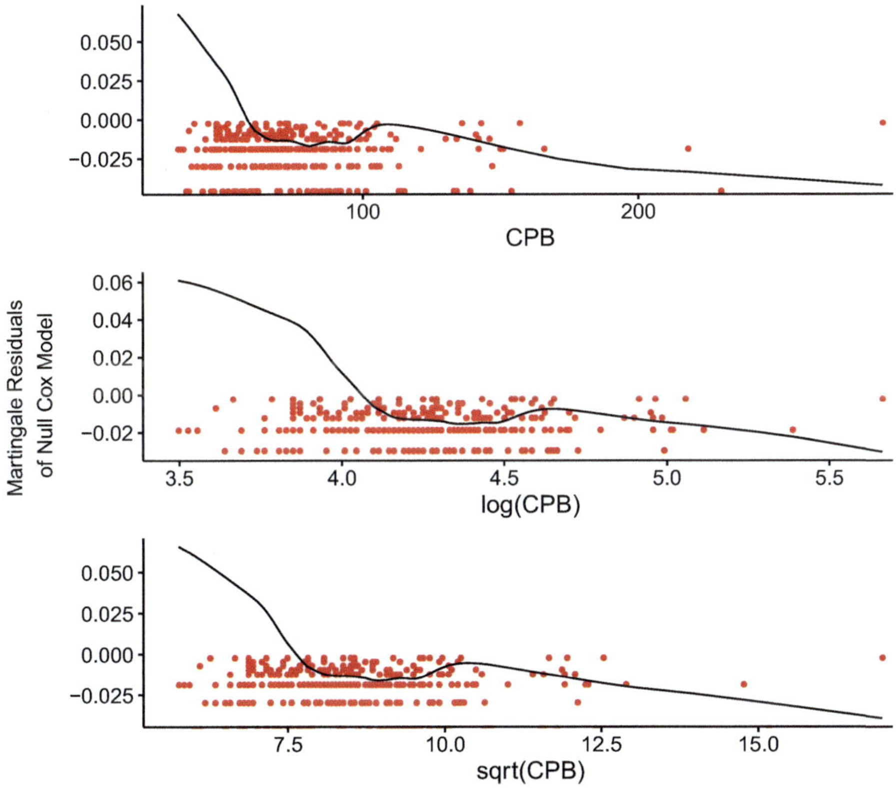

Fig. 11.16 Linear assumption

11.16 Proportionality Assumption Is not Met

In some circumstances the proportionality assumption (constant hazard ratio over time) is not met.

In plain words, there is a level of interaction between the explanatory variable (`Broccoli`) and time (`FUtime`). At a certain point in time the relationship between `Broccoli` and `FUtime` changes (an interaction occurs between `Broccoli` and `FUtime`). We may try to add more coefficients to *cover* the difference in risk change.

Understanding if the interaction term (`Broccoli * FUtime`) is significant is another way of testing a proportionality assumption, besides checking the Schoenfeld residuals. If the interaction term is not significant, then we may state that the assumption of proportionality is valid. It is very important to always plot the results and obtain a p-value. Some kind of non-proportional relationship and other proportional assumption can only be detected with a p-value.

To test for interaction we use the time transformation `tt` function.

```
> fit <- coxph(Surv(FUtime, FUmortality) ~ Broccoli + tt(Broccoli),
data=MMstat)
summary(fit)
```

As we see from Fig. 11.17, in this case the interaction between time-transformed `Broccoli` and time is associated with a non-significant p-value. Hence, the proportionality assumption for broccoli holds. This also confirms what the Schoenfeld residuals showed.

```
Call:
coxph(formula = Surv(FUtime, FUmortality) ~ Broccoli + tt(Broccoli),
    data = MMstat)

  n= 500, number of events= 58

                 coef exp(coef) se(coef)      z Pr(>|z|)
Broccoliy      2.1080    8.2321   2.9963  0.704    0.482
tt(Broccoli) -0.9825    0.3744   0.8870 -1.108    0.268

             exp(coef) exp(-coef) lower .95 upper .95
Broccoliy       8.2321     0.1215   0.02318  2923.656
tt(Broccoli)    0.3744     2.6712   0.06581     2.129

Concordance= 0.643  (se = 0.025 )
Likelihood ratio test= 16.62  on 2 df,   p=2e-04
Wald test            = 12.81  on 2 df,   p=0.002
Score (logrank) test = 14.75  on 2 df,   p=6e-04
```

Fig. 11.17 Testing for interaction

11.17 How to Choose Predictors

Selecting which covariates to include in a model is a very difficult task, especially when there are many of them. The first question to ask ourselves is *are we interested in the exact calculation of HR or instead in determining which covariates are the predictors of the outcome* (i.e., *these are the predictors of the event, whereas these others are not*)? In the latter case, the estimated size of the relationship's HR might be of secondary importance.

A method of automatic selection is *backward elimination.* As we learn from linear regression, backward elimination is less offensive. I describe in four steps below how to apply backward elimination:

1. First, we should fit the model containing all the chosen predictors. Those are either all the a priori ones (which we know from our experience may affect the outcome) or all the available ones (providing our dataset isn't too large). Then store the coefficients from the initial model. Obviously, we should keep in mind how frequent the outcomes of interest are. We should consider to fit one covariate (explanatory variable) for every ten events (i.e. death). For the sake of practising, let's include four predictors `Broccoli`, `Age`, `Bleeding` and `Male` (Fig. 11.18):

```
   > fit <- coxph(Surv(FUtime, FUmortality) ~
Broccoli+Male+Age+Bleeding, data=mmstat)
   > summary(fit)
```

2. Remove all predictors whose p-values are above a pre-set threshold, typically the usual 0.05 or 0.1 or sometimes just the highest p-value. In this case we should remove `Broccoli`, since the associated p-value is 0.5.
3. Now we re-run the model without `Broccoli` and compare the new coefficients with the coefficients from the original model (Fig. 11.19):
4. The p-value associated with `Bleeding` is 0.1. We could choose to remove this covariate and re-run the model, until all p-values are significant (Fig. 11.20).

```
coxph(formula = Surv(FUtime, FUmortality) ~ Broccoli + Male +
    Age + Bleeding, data = mmstat)

  n= 456, number of events= 14

               coef exp(coef)  se(coef)      z Pr(>|z|)
Broccoliy -0.385763  0.679932  0.683152 -0.565   0.5723
Male1     -1.207665  0.298894  0.723167 -1.670   0.0949 .
Age        0.579836  1.785745  0.126036  4.601 4.21e-06 ***
Bleeding  -0.003132  0.996873  0.001855 -1.689   0.0913 .
---
```

Fig. 11.18 Cox regression analysis output: removing the not significant variables

```
Call:
coxph(formula = Surv(FUtime, FUmortality) ~ Male + Age + Bleeding,
    data = mmstat)

  n= 456, number of events= 14

                coef exp(coef)  se(coef)       z Pr(>|z|)
Male1    -1.427872  0.239819  0.630115 -2.266   0.0234 *
Age       0.581443  1.788618  0.126920  4.581 4.62e-06 ***
Bleeding -0.003137  0.996868  0.001936 -1.620   0.1052
---
```

Fig. 11.19 Re-running the model after having removed the not significant variables

```
Call:
coxph(formula = Surv(FUtime, FUmortality) ~ Male + Age, data = mmstat)

  n= 456, number of events= 14

         coef exp(coef) se(coef)      z Pr(>|z|)
Male1 -1.2862    0.2763   0.6206 -2.073   0.0382 *
Age    0.6084    1.8375   0.1313  4.632 3.62e-06 ***
---
```

Fig. 11.20 Obtaining a model with only significant variables

Now we have a model with only two covariates, with significant p-values.

Importantly, the coefficients haven't changed much from the original model. The coefficient for male shifted from 0.29 (initial model) to 0.23, final model. The coefficient for Age shifted from 1.7 (initial model) to 1.8 (final model). If, however, we have a predictor whose coefficient has changed significantly, then we need to find the covariates that we removed and which are *correlated* with the affected predictor. We can explore that by adding back in one of the removed variables at a time, until the affected predictor's coefficient is back to its original value or thereabouts. In this scenario, we need to keep the removed variable in the model.

Let's make an example. Suppose that `Bleeding` is retained (original model with HR = 1.6, p = 0.05) but `Broccoli` is removed because it is not statistically significant (original model HR = 1.08, p = 0.20). But when we remove `Bleeding` from the original model, the HR for `Bleeding` changes from 1.6 to 1.9. This shift in HR is probably big enough to be worried about. Hence, we add `Broccoli` back in, and the original HR for `Bleeding` is restored. Importantly, we need to keep both `Bleeding` and `Broccoli` in the final model.

Correlation between variables is ignored by the stepwise procedure, which is why stepwise can be misleading and unreliable.

How big a shift in HR should cause worry? Unfortunately, this is arbitrary. Perhaps, anything less than 0.05 (i.e. a change from HR = 1.20 to HR = 1.24) is not significant. It depends sometimes on the context. For example, for important context of epidemiology (risk/decision making), even small changes in HR should be acknowledged.

Ultimately, once we decide the final model, we should check the residuals.

11.18 Conclusions

Kaplan-Meier, log-rank test and Cox regression models are widely used in time-to-event analysis. In this chapter we used survival function, visualised with the Kaplan-Meier model to plot the survival probability for `Broccoli=='y'` vs `Broccoli=='n'` groups. However, we did not notice significant differences since the log-rank test was not significant. Our Cox proportional regression model was undermined by the scarcity of events (*death*); hence, limited numbers of covariates were included in the final model. We concluded that in this simulation study, a broccoli dietary regimen is not associated with improved survival.

Further Readings

Barraclough H, Simms L, Govindan R. Biostatistics primer: what a clinician ought to know: hazard ratios. J Thorac Oncol. 2011;6(6):978–82. https://doi.org/10.1097/JTO.0b013e31821b10ab. Erratum in: J Thorac Oncol. 2011 Aug;6(8):1454.

Bland JM, Altman DG. Survival probabilities (the Kaplan-Meier method). BMJ. 1998;317(7172):1572. https://doi.org/10.1136/bmj.317.7172.1572.

Bland JM, Altman DG. The logrank test. BMJ. 2004;328(7447):1073. https://doi.org/10.1136/bmj.328.7447.1073.

Cox DR. Regression models and life-tables. J R Stat Soc Series B Stat Methodol. 1972;34(2):187–202.

Kleinbaum DG, Klein M. The cox proportional hazards model and its characteristics. In: Survival analysis. Statistics for biology and health. New York, NY: Springer; 2012.

Ogundimu EO, Altman DG, Collins GS. Adequate sample size for developing prediction models is not simply related to events per variable. J Clin Epidemiol. 2016;76:175–82. https://doi.org/10.1016/j.jclinepi.2016.02.031. Epub 2016 Mar 8

Rebernick RJ, Bell HN, Wakeam E. Survival analyses: a statistical review for surgeons. Semin Thorac Cardiovasc Surg. 2022;34(4):1388–94. https://doi.org/10.1053/j.semtcvs.2022.01.001.

Rich JT, Neely JG, Paniello RC, Voelker CC, Nussenbaum B, Wang EW. A practical guide to understanding Kaplan-Meier curves. Otolaryngol Head Neck Surg. 2010;143(3):331–6. https://doi.org/10.1016/j.otohns.2010.05.007.

Spruance SL, Reid JE, Grace M, Samore M. Hazard ratio in clinical trials. Antimicrob Agents Chemother. 2004;48(8):2787–92. https://doi.org/10.1128/AAC.48.8.2787-2792.2004.

Weng SW, Liao CC, Yeh CC, Chen TL, Lane HL, Lin JG, Shih CC. Risk of epilepsy in stroke patients receiving acupuncture treatment: a nationwide retrospective matched-cohort study. BMJ Open. 2016;6(7):e010539. https://doi.org/10.1136/bmjopen-2015-010539.

Chapter 12
Propensity Score Matching

Propensity Score Matching

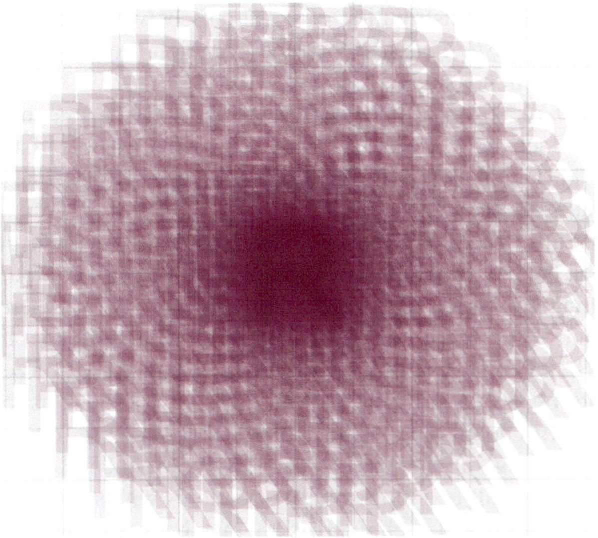

12.1 Software and R-Packages Required for This Chapter

If you haven't already, you need to download and install base-R and R-studio as set out in Chap. 2 under the heading "Downloading "R" and R-studio".

The relevant R-packages needed for this chapter are:

- MatchIt—it can be downloaded at:
- http://tidyverse.tidyverse.org
- tableone—it can be downloaded at:
- https://github.com/kaz-yos/tableone

M. Moscarelli, *Biostatistics With 'R': A Guide for Medical Doctors*,
https://doi.org/10.1007/978-3-031-33073-5_12

12.2 Where to Download the Example Dataset and Script for This Chapter

If you haven't already downloaded the supplementary dataset named `MMstat.csv` created as a practical example for use throughout this book, you will find it at the link that follows. The script for this chapter named `Chapter 12. Propensity score.R` can also be found and downloaded at the following link:

https://github.com/mmlondon77/Biobook.git

12.3 Matching and Propensity Score Matching

In randomised trials, the distribution of covariates between treated and control is balanced due to *stochastic balance* (the randomisation process). This process does not apply to observational studies.

In the context of observational studies, subjects in the treatment and control groups may in fact show several different baseline characteristics. Therefore, dissimilarities in outcomes may reflect the differences in baseline characteristics than a true treatment effect.

To overcome this issue, it is possible to match each subject in the treatment group with a subject in the control group, with comparable baseline confounders. We may achieve matching by one-to-one matching (*pair matching*), whereby we match exactly one control subject to one treated subject, or many to one, matching some fixed number (K) of control subjects to each treated subject (e.g. $K=3$, three-to-one matching). With regard to variables, we can use many of them, as long as they are meaningful and with no missing values, otherwise we can use just a few.

However, matching on the basis of several confounders can be a complex procedure and may result in a limited pool of patients with similar characteristics.

An alternative statistical technique is to match on the basis of the propensity score.

There are four propensity score-based methods. In this chapter I cover only propensity score *matching* (PSM).

The concept of PSM was introduced by Rosenbaum and Rubin as far back as 1983, in a paper published in Biometrika titled "The Central Role of the Propensity Score in Observational Studies for Causal Effects". PSM attempts to estimate the effect of a treatment (in our case scenario `Broccoli`) by accounting for the covariates that *predict* receiving the treatment. In other words, the aim of PSM is to match treated subjects (e.g. subjects from `Broccoli=='y'`) and control subjects (e.g. subjects from `Broccoli=='n'`) on their covariates (i.e. on the set of covariates that are identified as sufficient to control for confounding, as outlined previously in the book).

PSM is a specific kind of matching technique; again it accounts for the covariates that *predict* receiving the treatment and is derived from a logistic regression model (*distance on the propensity score*).

There are two main common types of PSM: the *nearest-neighbour matching* and *optimal matching.*

This chapter essentially covers the *nearest-neighbour* (greedy) matching.

12.4 Distance and Caliper

There are two important concepts for matching, one is *distance* and the other is *caliper.*

Distance is a metric of closeness; it tells how similar two covariates are to each other. The type of distance we select determines the type of matching. For PSM, distance is derived from a logistic regression model (probability of receiving a treatment, based on certain covariates). In "R" the default is *glm*, for propensity scores estimated with logistic regression using *glm*.

Caliper is the maximum acceptable distance. After the best match, the algorithm matches the treated subject if the best match has a distance less than the caliper. A tight caliper is preferred when matches are easy to find (e.g. when there is little difference between exposed and unexposed subjects and there is a large pool of unexposed subjects from which to select). A looser caliper is preferred when matches are harder. Caliper allows an increase in the quality of matching. Matching with replacement is an alternative to caliper adjustment. However, the latter is the technique considered to result in less biases.

A caliper of 0.20 is equal to 0.20 SD of logit of the propensity score.

12.5 Greedy (Nearest-Neighbour) Matching

The greedy matching matches a treatment with a control with the smallest distance available. Before proceeding for the actual PSM, we want to analyse the covariate imbalance between the two groups at baseline level.

12.6 Covariates and Probabilities of Treatment, Before PSM Table

Let us return to the patients' baseline characteristics. We explained how to use the `tableone` package in Chap. 4 which covered *data types* and how to create tables (Fig. 12.1):

	Stratified by Broccoli				
	n	y	p	test	SMD
n	297	203			
Age (mean (SD))	62.82 (12.81)	63.83 (13.19)	0.392		0.078
Weight (mean (SD))	74.95 (13.72)	73.68 (14.14)	0.318		0.091
Height (mean (SD))	168.28 (9.31)	166.20 (9.01)	0.013		0.228
LVEF (mean (SD))	52.11 (8.65)	53.44 (7.02)	0.071		0.168
Creatinine (mean (SD))	0.89 (0.29)	0.88 (0.29)	0.629		0.044
Male = 1 (%)	139 (46.8)	85 (41.9)	0.319		0.099
Diabetes (%)			0.550		0.100
0	247 (83.2)	166 (81.8)			
1	39 (13.1)	32 (15.8)			
2	11 (3.7)	5 (2.5)			
COPD (%)			0.749		0.070
0	271 (91.2)	189 (93.1)			
1	19 (6.4)	10 (4.9)			
NA	7 (2.4)	4 (2.0)			
Aspirin = 1 (%)	217 (73.1)	112 (55.2)	<0.001		0.380
LOS (mean (SD))	15.34 (8.97)	13.77 (11.60)	0.314		0.151
CPB (mean (SD))	80.15 (32.63)	63.31 (17.11)	<0.001		0.647
CC (mean (SD))	44.78 (20.74)	35.39 (13.84)	<0.001		0.532
Bleeding (mean (SD))	581.70 (191.09)	475.38 (114.85)	<0.001		0.674
Mortality = 1 (%)	39 (13.1)	5 (2.5)	<0.001		0.406

Fig. 12.1 Unmatched table—patients' baseline characteristics and relevant perioperative outcomes

```
> varsToFactor<-c("Male","Diabetes","Mortality","Aspirin", "COPD")
> MMstat[varsToFactor] <- lapply(MMstat[varsToFactor], factor)
> vars<- c('Age', 'Weight', 'Height', 'LVEF', 'Creatinine', 'Male',
'Diabetes','COPD', 'Aspirin', 'LOS','CPB', 'CC', 'Bleeding',
'Mortality')
> tableOne <- CreateTableOne(vars = vars, strata = c("Broccoli"),
data = MMstat, includeNA = TRUE)
> print(tableOne, smd=TRUE)
```

As we have seen in previous chapters, with regard to patients' baseline characteristics (highlighted within the red square in Fig. 12.1), there are some imbalances between `Broccoli=='n'` and `Broccoli=='y'`. There are differences in terms of `Height` and most importantly in terms of `Aspirin`. The latter may heavily influence the outcomes. Let us for the moment ignore the last column on the right, the standardised mean difference that is a measure of *balance*.

Notably, there are many differences in terms of perioperative outcomes (`CPB` and `CC`) and hard postoperative outcomes such as `Mortality` and `Bleeding`. However, such differences might be attributed to different baseline characteristics rather than to an actual treatment effect. We then need to equalise the confounders.

12.7 After PSM Table

To practically conduct PSM we need:

- `Grouping variable`: a variable that specifies which group a case belongs to (in our example the grouping variable is `Broccoli`).
- `Matching variables`: the covariates (confounders) we would like to attempt to equalise the groups on. In our example, they are highlighted in red in Fig. 12.1.

I now describe step by step how to perform PSM, using both `MatchIt` and `tableone` packages.

Importantly, we will use glm model to calculate the propensity score, because we have a *dependent variable* (i.e. the `Broccoli` treatment) as opposed to an *outcome of interest* (e.g. `Mortality`):

STEP 1: remove missing values. "R" is very sensitive to missing values. This is a major carveout for PSM techniques. A dataset with missing values will result in a loss of much information and potential patients to match. In order to proceed, we must remove the missing values first. To do so, we will use the `na.omit( )` function and create a new dataset named `propMMstat`:

```
> propMMstat=as.data.frame(na.omit(MMstat))
```

PSM cannot be performed when there are missing values. Other approaches would be to use multiple imputation to fill the missing cells or inverse proportional weighting techniques. However, those are beyond the scope of this book.

STEP 2: convert the treatment to number (`0` and `1`) and back to factor. In our dataset, the observations of the broccoli variable are entered as `'y'` or `'n'`. However, for the sake of PSM, those must be converted to `0` and `1` and the broccoli variable coded as a factor as per the code below:

```
> propMMstat$Broccoli<-ifelse(propMMstat$Broccoli=='y', 1, 0)
> propMMstat$Broccoli<-as.factor(propMMstat$Broccoli)
```

STEP 3: calculate the propensity score. For the actual propensity score matching procedure, we need to use the `matchit` function. Note that we need to specify all the variables that we want to *equalise*. Also, we need to specify the method, in our case nearest matching `methods='nearest'`, the ratio `ratio=1` and possibly the caliper `caliper=0.2`.

```
> p<-matchit(Broccoli~Age+Male+Aspirin+Diabetes+Weight+Height+LVE
F+Creatinine+COPD, methods='nearest', ratio=1, caliper=0.2,
data=propMMstat)
```

The distance was not specified since `glm( )` is the default. Note that a less tight caliper would return a bigger pool of matched patients.

STEP 4: perform the match. The actual match is carried out with the `match.data( )` function:

```
> mm.prop<- match.data(p)
```

STEP 5: visualise the results. It is important to plot the matched and unmatched treated vs control to visualise the shape of their distributions. To do so we will use the `plot( )` function (Fig. 12.2):

```
> plot(p, type = "jitter", col='darkgreen')
> plot(p, type = "hist")
```

The central part of Fig. 12.2 depicts the distribution of the matched treated vs matched control units. The shape of the distributions looks similar. The upper and the lower part of Fig. 12.2 depicts the distributions of the unmatched treated vs unmatched control units. Few treated units were not matched (upper part of the panel), while many control units were left unmatched (lower panel of the Fig. 12.3).

Another valid option is to plot, using histograms, the distributions of the raw treated and raw control units (Fig. 12.3 left side) and matched treated and matched control units (Fig. 12.3 right side). The matched distributions look more similar than the raw distributions.

STEP 6: create a post PSM table. Similar to the unmatched scenario, we now produce a table with the matched group. However, specific tests are needed to analyse the outcomes for the conditioned sample (Fig. 12.4):

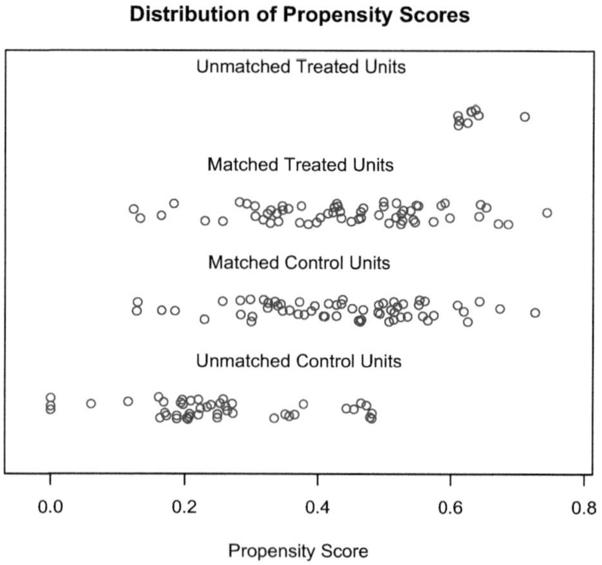

Fig. 12.2 Distribution of the matched and unmatched treated vs control units

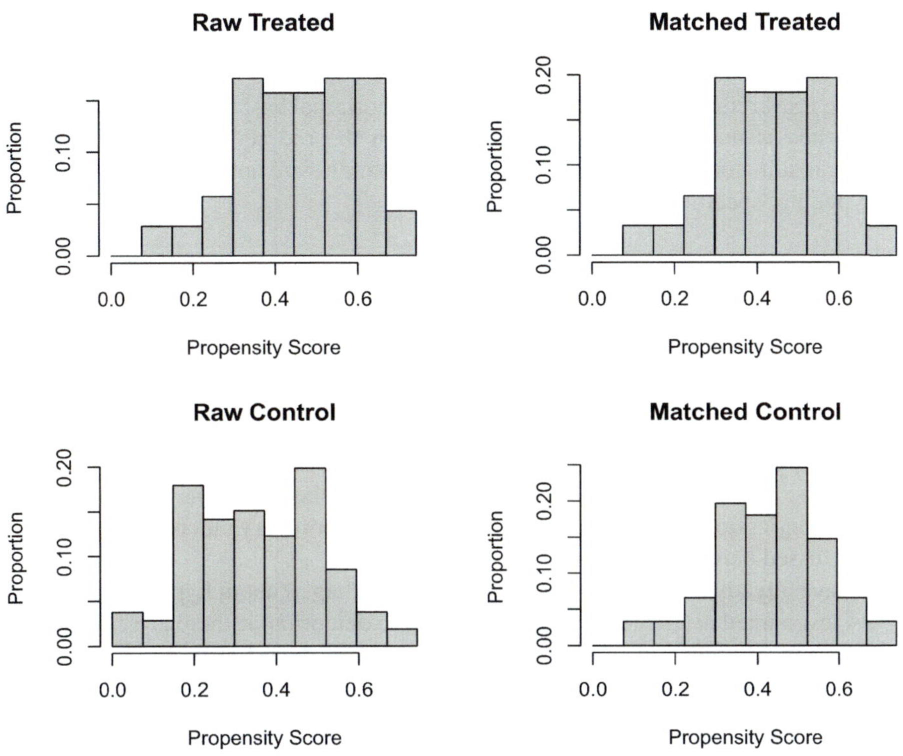

Fig. 12.3 Raw treated vs raw control units and matched treated vs matched control units—the shape of the histograms looks more similar and symmetric in the matched populations

	Stratified by Broccoli				
	0	1	p	test	SMD
n	61	61			
Age (mean (SD))	66.16 (12.33)	65.34 (12.30)	0.714		0.067
Weight (mean (SD))	71.87 (14.88)	72.77 (13.73)	0.729		0.063
Height (mean (SD))	165.05 (8.23)	164.75 (7.93)	0.841		0.037
LVEF (mean (SD))	53.69 (6.45)	53.41 (7.81)	0.830		0.039
Creatinine (mean (SD))	0.89 (0.33)	0.90 (0.27)	0.886		0.026
Male = 1 (%)	28 (45.9)	30 (49.2)	0.856		0.066
Diabetes = 1 (%)	12 (19.7)	12 (19.7)	1.000		<0.001
COPD = 1 (%)	2 (3.3)	2 (3.3)	1.000		<0.001
Aspirin = 1 (%)	32 (52.5)	32 (52.5)	1.000		<0.001

Fig. 12.4 PSM table—61 matched pairs were generated

```
> varsToFactor <- c("Male","Diabetes","Mortality","Aspi
rin", "COPD")
> mm.prop[varsToFactor] <- lapply(mm.prop[varsToFactor], factor)
> vars<- c('Age', 'Weight','Height', 'LVEF', 'Creatinine',
'Male', 'Diabetes','COPD', 'Aspirin')
> tableOne <- CreateTableOne(vars = vars, strata = c("Broccoli"),
```

```
data = mm.prop, includeNA = TRUE)
> print(tableOne, smd=TRUE)
```

The PSM returned 61 matched pairs (from an original basket of 500 patients). No imbalance is now detected (highlighted within the red square). The hypothesis testing results for the outcomes of the matched samples are not reported as yet, since they require specific tests.

12.8 Estimate the Treatment Effect in the Conditioned Sample

Matched data should be analysed using specific procedures for matched analyses, such as paired t-tests for continuous variables and McNemar's test for binary outcomes. Conditional logit or mixed effect (matched pairs as random effect) logistic regression (*doubly robust*) can also be used for binary outcomes but will not be discussed here.

I have already covered the paired `t.test` in Chap. 8 about hypothesis testing.

A test named `mcnemar.test()` is used to determine if there is a statistically significant difference in proportions between paired data. Let us for the moment produce a table with results from the matched samples (Fig. 12.5):

```
> vars2 <- c('LOS','CPB', 'CC', 'Bleeding', 'Mortality')
> tableOne <- CreateTableOne(vars = vars2, strata =
c("Broccoli"), data = mm.prop, test=FALSE)
> print(tableOne, smd=F)
```

Let us understand with a paired t-test if there are significant differences in bleeding between the matched groups (Fig. 12.6):

```
                        Stratified by Broccoli
                         0                1
  n                          61               61
  LOS (mean (SD))         13.64 (9.14)     14.66 (12.13)
  CPB (mean (SD))         78.49 (41.61)    60.08 (13.37)
  CC (mean (SD))          42.05 (22.09)    33.77 (10.96)
  Bleeding (mean (SD)) 565.44 (206.52) 453.10 (114.38)
  Mortality = 1 (%)          10 (16.4)         2 (3.3)
```

Fig. 12.5 Outcome of the matched pairs—the estimate of treatment effect needs to be evaluated with a paired t-test or McNemar's test

```
        Paired t-test

data:  propbroccoliy$Bleeding and propbroccolin$Bleeding
t = -3.4879, df = 60, p-value = 0.0009177
```

Fig. 12.6 Estimate of treatment effect, paired t-test

```
        McNemar's Chi-squared test with continuity correction

data:  Mc
McNemar's chi-squared = 33.391, df = 1, p-value = 7.536e-09
```

Fig. 12.7 Estimate of treatment effect, McNemar's test for binary outcome

```
> propbroccoliy<-mm.prop[mm.prop$Broccoli=='1',]
> propbroccolin<-mm.prop[mm.prop$Broccoli=='0',]
> t.test(propbroccoliy$Bleeding,propbroccolin$Bleeding,
paired=TRUE)
```

And perform for binary outcome the `mcnemar.test()` (Fig. 12.7):

```
> Mc<-table(mm.prop$Mortality, mm.prop$Broccoli)
> mcnemar.test(Mc)
```

`Mortality` and `Bleeding` remained significantly lower in the `Broccoli` group. Additionally, it must be noted that the operation times (`CPB` and `CC`) were significantly lower in the `Broccoli` group.

It is also important to note that the PSM could not control for `CPB` and `CC`. Those are *outcomes* rather the baseline covariates that could have influenced the choice of giving or not giving the broccoli dietary regimen to patients. Confounders should be measured/observed *before* the treatment is given.

With this in mind, since `CPB` and `CC` may affect both `Bleeding` and `Mortality`, the causal relationship between `Broccoli`, `Bleeding` and `Mortality` remains undetermined.

12.9 Doubly Robust Assessment

At this stage, data can also be analysed using a standard regression in the matched sample, which includes a treatment indicator and the variables used in the propensity score model (double robust) (Fig. 12.8):

```
> doubly<glm(Mortality~Broccoli+Age+Male+Aspirin+Diabetes+Weight+
Height+LVEF+Creatinine+COPD+CC
+CPB, family='binomial',data=mm.prop)#conducting the regression
model in the matched sample as double robust method.
> summary(doubly)
```

From the output of the table in Fig. 12.8, even in the `mm.prop` matched sample, `Broccoli` remained an independent predictor for `Mortality` (p=0.002), with a positive effect in reducing the 30-day post-operative mortality.

```
Coefficients:
              Estimate Std. Error z value Pr(>|z|)
(Intercept)  3.0154643  7.6018783   0.397   0.6916
Broccoli1   -2.5903276  0.8600575  -3.012   0.0026 **
Age         -0.0316351  0.0248330  -1.274   0.2027
Male         0.3276408  0.6423957   0.510   0.6100
Aspirin      0.7727507  0.7089281   1.090   0.2757
Diabetes     0.3292815  0.6207983   0.530   0.5958
Weight      -0.0033842  0.0287653  -0.118   0.9063
Height      -0.0005339  0.0476436  -0.011   0.9911
LVEF        -0.0067236  0.0416757  -0.161   0.8718
Creatinine  -0.2859101  1.3376136  -0.214   0.8307
COPD         2.2367995  1.6222367   1.379   0.1679
CC           0.0100318  0.0335023   0.299   0.7646
CPB         -0.0357348  0.0263748  -1.355   0.1755
```

Fig. 12.8 Doubly robust assessment, applying regression on the matched dataset

12.10 Assessing the Balance

The standardised difference is a metric of how the match/PSM works (balance after match).

Specifically, a standardised mean difference is the difference in means between groups, divided by the pooled standard deviation:

$$\text{smd} = \frac{\bar{X}\,\text{treatment} - \bar{X}\,\text{control}}{\sqrt{\dfrac{s^2\text{treatment} + s^2\text{control}}{2}}}$$

Basically, we compute a difference in means in standard deviation units (scaled difference). The smd is calculated for each covariate and does not depend on a sample size. As a rule of thumb:

- smd < 0.1: adequate balance
- smd = 0.1–0.2: not too alarming
- smd > 0.2: significant imbalance

Standardised differences are reported in the table pre- and post-matching. In our simulation, all the covariates after PSM have a smd < 0.1, suggesting a good performance of the matching.

The other way to check for balance after match is to perform hypothesis testing and look at the p-values between the two groups (e.g. test for a difference in means between treated and controls for each covariate). The drawback of the latter approach is that p-values are dependent on sample size; hence, a large sample size would return significant p-values for small differences. To show smd in the tables, we add the `print(tableOne, smd=TRUE)` command.

12.11 Conclusions

Given the nature of our study (cohort study type by definition with no stochastic balance), a statistical method to equalise the confounder is needed to reduce the selection bias.

The propensity score is the probability for a subject to receive a treatment, conditional on a set of certain baseline confounders (or characteristics). Propensity score is commonly estimated using logistic regression.

There are four propensity score-based methods. In this chapter we described the propensity score *matching* (PSM). There are also two types of PSM, which I described the nearest-neighbour (or greedy) matching. Also, a caliper adjustment was used to increase the quality of matching.

Further Readings

Austin PC. The performance of different propensity score methods for estimating marginal odds ratios. Stat Med. 2007;26:3078–94.

Benedetto U, Head SJ, Angelini GD, Blackstone EH. Statistical primer: propensity score matching and its alternatives. Eur J Cardiothorac Surg. 2018;53:1112–7.

Qu Y, Lipkovich I. Propensity score estimation with missing values using a multiple imputation missingness pattern (MIMP) approach. Stat Med. 2009;28:1402–14.

Randolph JJ, Falbe K, Manuel AK, Balloun JL. A step-by- step guide to propensity score matching in R. Pract Assess Res Evaluation. 2014;19(18).

Rosenbaum PR, Rubin DB. The central role of the propensity score in observational studies for causal effects. Biometrika. 1983;70(1):41–55.

Rubin DB, Thomas N. Matching using estimated propensity scores: relating theory to practice. Biometrics. 1996;52:249–64.

GPSR Compliance

The European Union's (EU) General Product Safety Regulation (GPSR) is a set of rules that requires consumer products to be safe and our obligations to ensure this.

If you have any concerns about our products, you can contact us on ProductSafety@springernature.com

In case Publisher is established outside the EU, the EU authorized representative is:

Springer Nature Customer Service Center GmbH
Europaplatz 3
69115 Heidelberg, Germany

Batch number: 10726060

Printed by Printforce, the Netherlands